So you've got pelvic pain... here's how to manage it.

A musculoskeletal approach to relieving persistent pelvic pain for men and women

PETER DORNAN

AM DIP PHTY, FASMF

www.
AUSTRALIANACADEMICPRESS
.com.au

First published in 2014 as Pelvic Pain: A musculoskeletal approach for treatment
This edition published 2019
Australian Academic Press Group Pty. Ltd.

www.australianacademicpress.com.au

A catalogue record for this
book is available from the
National Library of Australia

So you've got pevlic pain ... Here's how to manage it.

ISBN 9781925644272 (paperback)
ISBN 9781925644289 (ebook)

Disclaimer
Every effort has been made in preparing this work to provide information based on accepted stan-
dards and practice at the time of publication. The publisher, however, makes no warranties of any
kind of psychological outcome relating to use of this work and disclaims all responsibility or liability
for direct or consequential damages resulting from any use of the material contained in this work.

Publisher: Stephen May

Copy editing: Naomi Sysak

Cover design: Luke Harris, Working Type Studio

Typesetting: Australian Academic Press

Printing: Lightning Source

Contents

Acknowledgments...v

About the Author...vi

Introduction
So, you've got pelvic pain I

    A New Approach...6

    Summary..13

Chapter 1
Anatomy, Biomechanics and Pathology..15

    The Pelvic Girdle...15

    The Sacroiliac Joint...15

    The Pudendal Nerve...18

    Filling and Emptying the Bladder..24

    Nerve Supplies to Anal Sphincter and the Rectum....................................26

    A Discussion on Pain after Orgasm and Ejaculation..................................31

    Overview of Nerve Distribution to Major Anatomical Areas..................34

    Erectile Function...35

Chapter 2
Musculoskeletal Assessment...37

    Patient History...38

    Physical Assessment...42

Chapter 3

Treatment 45

    Releasing the Restrictions Maintaining the Innominate in an Incorrect
    Position on the Sacrum...45

    Maintaining correct lumbar posture 52

    Managing flare-ups: Neural Hypersensitivity 60

    A Word Here on Smudging..63

    Chronic Pain Management 65

References..71

Acknowledgments

A book of this nature relies heavily on the support of not only members of the medical profession, but also on the many sufferers, survivors and patients who have shared their problems and experiences with me. The collective courage, humility and support by individual members continue to inspire me.

I would particularly like to acknowledge the role of my colleagues from the Centre of Clinical Research Excellence (CCRE) Spine at the University of Queensland, Drs Michel Coppieters, Paul Hodges, Gwen Jull and Ruth Sapsford. I am extremely grateful to Michel, my supervisor and co-author during four years of research at the Centre. I am also extremely grateful to Dr Bruce Mitchell, a Sports and Interventional Pain Physician from Metro Spinal Clinic in Melbourne.

I would particularly like to pay tribute to the role of my friend and urologist, Dr Les Thompson, for his insight and consistent encouragement and direction over the last fifteen years with this project. I am indebted also to the many other urologists, radiologists, other specialists, doctors and physiotherapists who have assisted me to further my understanding in this area, particularly special members of the Women's and Men's Pelvic Health Special Interest Group of the Australian Physiotherapy Association.

A special accolade also goes to my dedicated Office Manager, Carol Marchant, whose patience and assistance in both typing and compiling the many drafts of this manuscript has been invaluable.

I wish also to express my gratitude to the many caring friends and health professionals I have met both internationally and locally, especially through the International Pelvic Pain Society (IPPS) and Professor Thierry Van Caillie's Women's Health and Research Institute at the University of New South Wales.

Finally, I would like to thank my wife, Dimity, for being my continual support system and my tireless cheer squad leader when problems seemed insurmountable.

About the Author

For 52 years, Peter Dornan has been a physiotherapist in the fields of sports medicine and manipulative therapy, working with many international sporting teams, including being the inaugural physiotherapist for the Australian national rugby union team, the Australian national rugby league team, the Queensland rugby union team, and the Australian cricket team. For his achievements, he was awarded the Commemorative 2000 Australian Sports Medal. He is also a passionate Men's Health activist. In 1997, Peter created a forum for men and their partners to gain support and be better informed in matters relating to prostate cancer. In 1998, he was influential in forming the Prostate Cancer Foundation of Australia.

Peter has also been freelance writing for many years and has written two books on sporting injuries, one on prostate cancer, (*Conquering Incontinence*) and four military books (*The Silent Men*, an account of the Kokoda Track Campaign, *Nicky Barr — An Australian Air Ace*, *The Last Man Standing*, an account of the Tobruk and El Alamein Campaigns, and *Diving Stations*, an inspiring story of one of the most successful submarine commanders of World War II).

In 2002, Peter was appointed as a Member of the General Division of the Order of Australia (AM).

Peter is married to Dimity Dornan (AO), a Speech Pathologist, who is the Founder and Executive Director of 'Hear and Say', a world-wide charity which teaches babies who are deaf to listen and to speak. They have two adult children, Melissa and Roderick.

For further information see www.peterdornanphysio.com.au

So, you've got pelvic pain…

This book is written as an update, and presents a wider perspective, for my first book on pelvic pain, *Pelvic Pain: A musculoskeletal Approach to treatment*. Ultimately, it is written for patients who have a specific variety of pelvic pain; pain or other symptoms related to the pelvis that does not respond to specialist intervention by physicians, urologists, gynaecologists, gastroenterologists and pain management specialists.

It is also written for health professionals who are interested in pelvic pain. It will be particularly useful for physiotherapists. If the patient has any of the following conditions, ones that have resisted traditional medical treatment, it is possible they may well have a musculoskeletal cause.

- Pain (or altered sensations) in the scrotum, penis (shaft or the tip of the glans), labia, vulva, vagina, perineum and pelvic floor region, anorectal region, low abdomen, bladder or prostate region or groin. These 'altered sensations' may be described as stabbing, numbness, tingling, buzzing, electric, deep ache, burning, lumpy feeling or pinching. Patients may report sensations that their pelvic anatomy is altered or missing, such as feeling that the anus or another object is drawn up inside the bowel. The pain can be triggered either from a sudden physical movement or event relating to pelvic dysfunction or if the condition is chronic, from a heightened sensitivity to palpation. It can also be evoked subtly over a long period of time, such as from extended periods of incorrect sitting.

- Dysuria (painful or difficult urination), irritable bowel and/or irritable bladder syndromes, urgency or frequency incontinence — faecal or urinary, pain or difficulty during or after voiding — either defecation or micturition.

- Sexual and erectile dysfunctions including impotence, persistent genital arousal (without desire) and priapism (persistent erections). Pain during or after intercourse, ejaculation or orgasm.

- Changes in skin temperature and/or sensory changes in skin, itchiness, redness in lower abdomen areas, groin, thighs, anus or genitals, often producing intolerance to tight underclothes and certain cloth textures. The scrotum may appear blue or darker, shrink and draw up into the pelvis.

To articulate plausible explanations for persistent pelvic pain, a quick look at the medical literature, text books or 'Dr Google', (as most patients already have done) reveals the answer may well be complicated. Generally, authorities will agree the most consistent cause may be a complex interaction between the gastro-intestinal, genito-urinary, musculoskeletal, neurologic and endocrine systems, influenced by socio-cultural factors.

In fact, this is reinforced by the official definition of chronic pelvic pain (CPP) which was developed and accepted by the IASP (International Association for the study of Pain) Council in 2012.

Chronic pelvic pain is chronic or persistent pain perceived in structures related to the pelvis of either men or women. It is often associated with negative cognitive, behavioural, sexual and emotional consequences as well as with symptoms suggestive of lower urinary tract, sexual, bowel, pelvic floor or gynaecological dysfunction. It is often characterised by sudden and unpredictable 'flare ups', lasting anywhere from a few hours to a few days or longer.

A significant number of patients present under the idiopathic (which means we don't really know), non-infective and non-bacterial classifications. During the diagnostic process, specialist medical attention would have considered such common pelvic pain conditions as interstitial cystitis, prostatitis, vulvodynia, endometriosis, cancers and prolapses, ano-rectal dysfunction, proctalgia fugax, pelvic floor muscle pain syndrome, obturator internus and piriformis syndromes, and neuropathic pain (nerve) syndromes. Specialists will uncover many more not-so-usual conditions.

A useful system, developed by three urologists from Cleveland Clinic (USA) in 2010, Shoskes, Nickel and Kattan, which reminds the Health Practitioner to consider all domains in the assessment and diagnosis of pelvic pain, is called the UPOINT approach*. UPOINT is an acronym which stands for:

U — Urinary dysfunction

P — Psychosocial (clinical depression, catastrophysizing, helplessness)

O — Organ specific changes (bladder, prostate, sex organs)

I — Infection (urine culture, prostate expression)

N — Neurogenic or systemic dysfunction (pain outside the pelvis)

T — Tenderness — (pelvic tissues, pain with palpation, spasm)

If this system reveals a potential diagnosis and fails to respond to traditional medical treatment, it should be considered the patient may have a musculoskeletal cause.

Further, various types of pain must be considered — nociceptive (which arises from irritation of peripheral sensory nerves — from fractures, sprains or bruises after a fall, perhaps), visceral (from visceral organs, bladder etc. — a disease, perhaps), functional (movement related) and neuropathic, which is the result of injury or malfunction in the peripheral or central nervous system. I am going to concentrate on this last condition – neuropathic pain.

Neuropathic pain is defined as pain due to nerve damage and/or pain arising as a direct consequence of a lesion or disease affecting the somatosensory system. (Treede et al., 2008)[1]. The dominant and particular nerve involved here with the pelvis is the **Pudendal Nerve,** but there are others.

Many pelvic and perineal pains are now categorised as pudendal neuralgia. However, as has already been stated, making such a diagnosis is not easy (and may not be accurate) as many nerves may be involved, from both somatic and autonomic nervous systems. As well, many mechanisms may be involved including damage to other anatomical structures.

In many cases, I contend there may be a musculoskeletal component involved with the cause of these symptoms. Often a clue for this involvement is that the pelvic pain symptoms are regularly associated with a history of low back pain, with or without groin, buttocks and leg symptoms. They are often initiated by sitting or sitting can make them worse. Cycling can be a common cause.

The pudendal nerve supplies each and all of these aforementioned anatomical structures and regions which can give rise to all the symptoms mentioned

---

* From: Guidelines on Chronic Pelvic Pain, D.Engelfa et al., European Assoc of Urology.

in the opening paragraphs, and it monitors, influences and is associated with their individual functions. The nerve is a key component in providing sensations that range from pleasure to pain. If this nerve is compromised in any way, from its origin to anywhere along its course, it can produce the potential to give rise to any, or a combination of all, of the above symptoms, including paresthesia and pain. The diagnosis then is **Pudendal Neuropathy**. There has been some mystery involved with this diagnosis. We should search further.

Pudendal Neuropathy encompasses all diseases of the pudendal nerve and may or may not involve pain. The term **Pudendal Neuralgia** (PN) is a sub heading of Pudendal Neuropathy and describes pain of a severe throbbing or stabbing character in the course of the nerve. Pudendal neuralgia is a neuropathic pain condition involving inflammation and dysfunctional firing of the nerve due to trauma or disease. The nerve can become sensitised (over stimulated) and send out heightened signals to the genitals and associated systems.

The term **Pudendal Nerve Entrapment** (PNE) is defined as a focal nerve lesion produced by constriction or mechanical distortion of the nerve anywhere along its course. It can give rise to symptoms of pudendal neuralgia, however, pudendal neuralgia can also result from other causes.

Because the diagnosis PNE implies the nerve may be irrevocably entrapped or caught somewhere, it gives the impression surgery may be the only means of treatment. In reality, only a small minority of patients will have this situation. It is therefore important a clear diagnosis is made. A pudendal nerve block can sometimes ascertain if the pudendal nerve is involved.

In 1990, Labat et al.,[2] stated that anaesthetic pudendal nerve blocks, when used as a diagnostic test, were considered positive if there was total relief of pain when sitting within one hour of infiltration.

More recently, in 2007, Labat et al.[3], a Frenchman, states that the diagnosis of PNE is essentially clinical. A working party has validated a set of simple diagnostic criteria, the Nantes Criteria. The five essential signs and symptoms are:

1. Pain in the anatomical territory of the pudendal nerve.
2. Pain is worsened by sitting.
3. The patient is not woken at night by pain.
4. No objective sensory loss on clinical examination.
5. Positive anaesthetic pudendal nerve block.

However, since then, it appears one of the most valid means to diagnose actual entrapment at present is with Magnetic Resonance Neurography, (MRN). [Simply, MRN is an MRI of a nerve].

Aaron Filler[4], a surgeon from California, has documented four possible different locations of entrapment, by MRN investigation. On a series of 189 patients which were diagnosed with PNE, the four categories he found were:

1. Entrapment exclusively at the level of the piriformis muscle in the sciatic notch only. (2%)

2. Entrapment at the level of the ischial spine and sacrotuberous ligament. (5%)

3. Entrapment in the Alcock (or pudendal) canal on the medial surface of the obturator internus muscle. (80%)

4. Entrapment at the distal branches of the pudendal nerve. (13%)

There may now be other methods to make this diagnosis clearer. Professor Thierry Vancaille, a Gynaecologist and Pain Specialist from the University of New South Wales, reported from a 2011 'Pudendalhope' site,(support site on the net), that by using dynamic fluoroscopy, a radio-opaque dye is used to localise Alcock's Canal and the infra-piriformis canal. He states he is now developing a technique to combine MRI and the neurography to try and gain a clearer understanding of the anatomy. He also reports that a single injection of a pudendal nerve block results in a substantial improvement in at least 40% of patients.

However, in 2003, Dr Jerome Weiss[5] reported that Professor Roger Robert, a neurosurgeon in Nantes, France, found in his surgical patients, the source of the entrapment was at the sacrospinous ligament in 58%, and/or the sacrotuberous ligament in 69%, and often included the falciform process of the sacrotuberous ligament in 42%.

The troubling potential prognosis for a compressed or entrapped nerve relates to the pathophysiology involving ischaemia of blood vessels supplying the nerve. Subsequent collagen deposition and fibrosis (scarring) can increase the intraneural pressure and can initiate a self-perpetuating cycle of pain causing neural hypersensitivity.

Importantly, a competent MRN which clears entrapment as a diagnosis can amount to a revelation which is often a liberating moment for these patients. It means they may now be able to confidently search for a more moderate form of treatment than surgery — and be patient when coping with the effects of hypersensitivity.

For the patient, at the initial consultation with their Health Professional, he or she may have considered the end point (or end structure) of that nerve to be the problem. That is, if the patient presents and complains of say, a painful scrotum or vulva, he or she may be diagnosed as having a local condition such as an infected or inflamed testicle (orchialgia) or vulvadynia. The patient may indeed be treated for this diagnosis and perhaps be prescribed antibiotics. This can often give temporary relief as it is known that some antibiotic (anti-bacterial) agents can have a therapeutic anti-inflammatory effect; the precise mechanisms remain to be elucidated. The patient may also be given relieving medications, anti-inflammatories or surgery — in fact, surgical removal of a testicle, or a hysterectomy, (to relieve the pain) is not uncommon. The patient may also be offered other physical interventions, such as injections of Marcaine, steroids, Botox, hyaluronaidase, and intraoperative placement of adhesiolytic agents, typically Seprafilm.

Further, integral with this diagnosis, long term distress, caused by chronic symptoms, regularly is associated with co-morbidities of depression, anxiety and fear. Couple this with minimally or temporarily effective treatments given by a plethora of physicians and therapists, and the loss of quality of life, can lead to cognitive decline. This situation is then often treated by anti-depressants.

All, or any, of these treatments, including the anti-depressants, may temporarily relieve the symptoms. However if the real cause is a compromise of the pudendal nerve, in any of its presentations, the relief may be short term. (Including for the patient with the removed testicle or hysterectomy). The patient may then have his/her diagnosis assigned into a different classification — **Chronic Pelvic Pain Syndrome** (CPPS). Chronic pain is defined as daily pain that continues for three months or more. There is a move to change this label to "Persistent Pelvic Pain Syndrome", implying that the word "chronic" may inhibit any treatment program.

I must reinforce there can be several nerves and systems involved with this diagnosis, which I will mention later, but for now, I want to concentrate on the pudendal nerve.

A New Approach

There are obviously many valid ways that the pudendal nerve can be compromised, such as from a disease process, during surgery or from a traumatic sporting or motor vehicle accident. However, clinically, I have observed that many of the above conditions (mentioned on pages 3 and 4) are often associated with pelvic girdle dysfunction involving the sacroiliac joint, which, as I shall explain, can compromise the pudendal nerve.

My argument therefore, is that many forms of persistent pelvic pain may have its origins in pelvic dysfunction which may lead to irritation of structures innervated by the nerve.

Some work has already been done by Physiotherapists from this angle. Stephanie Prendergast and Elizabeth Rummer[6] from the United States have charted a number of musculoskeletal impairments which can be associated with pudendal neuralgia. They list such conditions as pelvic floor dysfunction, connective tissue restrictions, myofascial trigger points, (particularly in the obturator internus muscle), muscle hypertonicity, altered neurodynamics, sacroiliac joint dysfunction and other structural/biomechanical abnormalities and central sensitisation.

They state that in the case of sacroiliac joint dysfunction, extreme or abnormal joint positions, such as pelvic rotations may result in increased tension on the ligaments through which the pudendal nerve passes. As a result, the ligaments may compress or shear the nerve and lead to inflammation, setting up the painful symptoms.

This concept then will introduce a specific perspective to managing these conditions; a musculoskeletal approach. This different strategy is often a conflicting, difficult and challenging notion to a patient who has had a reinforced belief that something must be wrong at the local end-site, for example with the testicle, vulva, prostate, bladder, rectum etc.

I am a Sports Physiotherapist with a strong experience of managing spinal and musculoskeletal conditions. What would I know of this? Let me explain briefly my involvement.

About fifteen years ago, an urologist friend of mine consulted me for treatment of a painful lower back with associated referred symptoms to his left shin. He sustained it by lifting weights and executing split squat exercises at the gym. It was a routine consultation for me. I was able to deliver a simple diagnosis and prescribe an uncomplicated treatment. I diagnosed him as having sustained a sprained sacroiliac joint where the innominate bone (colloquially known as the pelvic bone of the pelvis) had been forced into extreme posterior rotation on the sacrum (see Figure 8 on page 38).

I treated it by selecting an appropriate mobilisation technique and exercises. He phoned in next day to thank me and report that his back and shin pain was gone, and to his amazement, so was his scrotal pain. I wasn't aware that initially he had scrotal pain as he hadn't complained of it. In fact, patients never walk into a Physiotherapist at first contact and complain of scrotal pain or any of the previously mentioned pelvic symptoms — they will rightly go to their medical practitioner.

"What had I done?" he asked. "I've been to every urologist and specialist in Brisbane and couldn't find a cause or treatment. I was about to have surgery".

My friend confided he had several cases of patients who had presented with scrotal pain which had not responded to his treatment — he would send them to me. One of the first patients had a clinical diagnosis of prostatitis and had been on antibiotics for two years. However, after looking at all his pathology, the urologist found no evidence of any prostatic infection or other urological problem. Within two weeks of mobilising and exercise, the symptoms had resolved.

In fact, all the patients responded to this approach. My friend then challenged me, "You had better find out what you are doing and why you are getting results". Quick research revealed that the scrotum is supplied predominately by the pudendal nerve (although other nerves can be involved). I also found that the pudendal nerve supplies and controls most of the major organs and systems in the pelvic area. In fact, it supplies all of the areas involving the previously cited symptoms and functions. That set me off on a serious path of research and discovery.

I went back to the University of Queensland and studied with Michel Coppieters, a PhD Physiotherapist who specialises in neural pain. I then revisited the anatomy lab, and with another Physiotherapist, Dr Susan Mercer, dissected out the pudendal nerve and followed its course from its origin in the sacrum, at the base of the spine, to where it moves through the pelvis. We then examined its mechanics and relationship with the sacroiliac joint, the large joint which joins the sacrum to the pelvis. We then looked for possible reasons why damage to this joint could impact on the nerve, then, with this information, I fine-tuned my mobilising techniques and exercise program.

Quite simply, as I shall explain in the coming chapters, and as suggested by Prendergast and Rummers[6], I considered that if either of the flanking bones of the pelvis, that is, the innominates, (see Figure 8 on page 38) was rotated significantly on the sacrum, (injury from sport, work, lying heavily and incorrectly during surgery, or pregnancy or sitting incorrectly), a situation could indeed be set up where the pudendal nerve (and other sacral and lumbar nerves) could be compromised.

It is well accepted now that the nervous system slides and glides as we move. Broadly, as a result of this process, the pudendal nerve could be harmed through several possible mechanisms; compression, stretch, (creating what is known as altered nerve biomechanics) or entrapped between or around other anatomical structures. I proposed that any of these processes could potentially lead to the symptoms detailed at the beginning of this introduction.

A large part of this study was to establish the role that posture, in particular, sitting posture, and lumbar-pelvic mechanics played in causing and managing this condition. Long periods of incorrect sitting were found to be a consistent denominator in the cause, as well as exacerbating the symptoms. This was particularly so amongst workers who sit at computers all day, and with drivers, (taxis, couriers, tractors), and addicted television viewers. Importantly, this research revealed that more nerves than the pudendal nerve may be involved with this scenario.

The final important aspect to address was how to manage and treat hypersensitivity of the nerve. Without correctly identifying the cause of these symptoms, (and therefore addressing and treating the cause) continued repetitive stressing of the nerve, sometimes for years, has the potential to set up debilitating, over- reactive, inappropriate and complex pain cycles, (termed hypersensitivity).

In regards to complex pain cycles, I include several other points for completeness. It is worthwhile mentioning that some therapists consider that the same pudendal neuralgia symptoms could be triggered by viscero-somatic reactions set up by other disease processes in the pelvis. Such conditions as endometriosis, irritable bowel and irritable bladder syndromes, chronic bladder and kidney infections, medical interventions such as hysterectomy and prostatectomy, and conditions which arise from ovarian, uterine, vaginal, vulvi and labial areas, may all set up a painful viscero-somatic reflex. It can be seen in a diagram of the pudendal nerve map (see Figure 3a on page 19), that the pelvic splanchnic nerve (which carries the viscero-somatic nervous system), and the pudendal nerve, both emanate from S2, 3 and 4. It is speculated that this closeness may set up the prospect of "mutual influence" in the nerves.

There is some evidence that suggests that afferent stimuli arising from such a visceral disorder (of any of the above-mentioned conditions), through a process known as 'viscerosomatic convergence', can lead to sensory and motor changes in muscle, viscera, blood vessels and skin. These effects can be detected in particular areas of skin associated with the nerve roots of an inflamed branch of the pudendal nerve. This can lead to external tissue dysfunction and is known as subcutaneous panniculosis. These effects can also be detected in the presence of myofascial trigger points (sensitive focal points in the underlying muscle), although this concept is now being contested (see next paragraph).

Trained therapists tackle this reaction by applying manual myofacial trigger point release procedures, connective tissue massage and special skin rolling techniques on all sensitive and painful areas as previously stated. However, recently the evidence for the existence of trigger points and the effectiveness of myofascial muscle techniques have been challenged and the process is controversial. This point is further discussed in the final chapter, Chapter 3.

Along these lines, specially certified Physiotherapists, for some years, have practiced a form of therapy called *pelvic floor physical therapy*. The aim is to carry out targeted internal vaginal soft tissue manipulation, a massage, to relieve pelvic pain by accessing muscles which cannot be reached any other way. In the case of males with pelvic pain, the massage is typically performed through the anus. This form of therapy has been tested and found effective in several small studies.

In particular, physiotherapist Dr Rhonda Kotarinos, from Chicago, is one of the authors of a 2013 study, published in the Journal of Urology. Their study randomly assigned 81 women with pelvic floor tenderness and painful bladder syndrome to either 10 sessions of pelvic floor therapy or 10 sessions of full body massage.

Women who received the targeted pelvic floor physical therapy were more likely to respond to therapy, with 59 percent experiencing improvement in symptoms compared with 26 percent in the full body massage group.

Another suggested contributing factor in the multi-layered presentation and management of this condition targets anxiety as a stimulus for causing pelvic pain. This concept considers that in predisposed individuals, chronic stress reactions cause muscle spasm and pain. The state of chronic constriction creates pain-referring trigger points, reduced blood flow, and an inhospitable environment for the nerves, blood vessels and structures throughout the pelvic basin. This results in a cycle of pain, anxiety and tension. The Wise-Anderson Protocol[7] relies, among other techniques, on the central practice of attention training in relaxing the pelvic floor, the use of RSA (respiratory sinus arrhythmia) breathing, (being aware of your breathing rates) during Trigger Point Release, and further insights in the practise of Paradoxical Relaxation.

Keeping in mind the controversies just cited concerning the existence of trigger points, and the further discussion in Chapter 3 on chronic pain management, there has been research that does support the integration of myofascial trigger point release (if that is what is actually being released), and paradoxical relaxation training treatment of chronic pelvic pain syndrome in men. In the Journal of Urology in 2005 Anderson and colleagues[8] published a study which involved 138 men with CP/CPPS who had not responded to traditional treatment methods. The men were treated with trigger point release therapy once a week for four weeks and then biweekly for eight weeks. They also received paradoxical relaxation therapy for at least one month. The men completed daily practice sessions (each lasting one hour per day) for six months.

More than 50% of the men had a 25% or greater decrease in their pain or urinary scores, and 72% of the men reported moderate or marked improvement in their symptoms. Of the men who had at least 50% improvement, their pain decreased by 69% and their urinary symptoms declined by 80%.

Along these lines, recent research by psychologist Rachel Muller [9] and colleagues have recorded that the deliberate engagement in positive activities for 15 minutes one day a week for eight weeks has a significant effect on wellbeing and on pain symptoms. Choosing such activities as acts of kindness to others, expressing gratitude, savouring a positive experience and engaging in a challenging or absorbing task, study participants recorded significant benefits in pain intensity, pain control, pain catastrophising and life satisfaction.

Food and diet rarely have been considered to be a cause of pudendal neuralgia, however, there is some evidence that glucose intolerance and certain acidic foods can trigger the symptoms. Caffeine, alcohol, yeast and bacterial infections have also been known to sensitize (flare) the nerve. An interesting variant of this sensitivity is tingling in the teeth before urination during urinary urgency build up. These must be considered in the overall assessment plan. There is also evidence that an anti-inflammatory style diet can ease painful symptoms, such as a Mediterranean Diet. (See Chapter 3).

Another area of research opening now which has been shown to have an effect on causing chronic pain relates to survivors who had suffered abuse as a child. The Blue Knot Foundation puts this at one in every four Australians, including sexual, physical, emotional or neglect, a very high percentage. Childhood abuse can have profound physical health repercussions in adulthood.

Survivors of trauma may possess high sensitisation which can impact their tolerance for relatively minor stresses. They are virtually allergic to stressors, are often hypervigilant, waiting for the next assault. Often, their body is resilient to coping with trauma later in life. Repeated traumatic experiences in childhood can affect stress hormones, an effect which can carry through to adulthood.

Particularly for women with chronic pelvic pain. Researchers have often noted a link to some women being early victims of sexual abuse. More recent research seeks to identify a biological explanation for the correlation of the well-established link between childhood trauma, torture, accidents etc to poor health outcomes later in life, with a particular focus on the reactivity of the neuro-immune-endocrine system.

This relates to what is called allostatic overload, which is where a system is constantly in a state of trying to adjust to stresses and there is an impact on the functioning of those systems if the load gets too much. This is a valid view we have to keep looking at.

Once again, I mention these concepts for the sake of completeness. What is evident however is the high percentage of patients with CPPS who cannot be given a contributing etiology. Mathias et al (1996)[10] have stated, of nine million women in the United States who had been diagnosed with CPPS, (20% of these lasting more than a year in duration), only 39% had a confirmed diagnosis, so the majority had no obvious etiology. Similarly, approximately 95% of men diagnosed with chronic prostatitis do not have an infection. (Roberts et al., 1997)[11].

In fact, recent research has found that the diagnosis of prostatitis is mainly a myth. The first mention of treatment of prostatitis is from Dr J.S. Hughes' 1860 book on 'Diseases of the Prostate Gland'. His treatment consisted of leeches (to the perineum), blood-letting, ice cubes in the rectum and opiate suppositories. Nothing apparently changed much for a century until this diagnosis was reintroduced in 1968 after a study of six patients with pelvic pain. After a urinalysis the diagnosis of prostatitis was made and it stuck. The presenting symptoms of pain in the low abdomen, around the anus, groin or back, difficulty urinating and pain after urination is now generally attributed to a variation of pudendal neuralgia, not prostatitis, as it once was.

My research, which was published in the British Journal of Urology International Oct 2012[12] and my clinical experience, would suggest that as much as 95% of patients who present with these symptoms, and have been cleared of any urological, gynaecological or gastrointestinal cause, may be associated with **lumbar-pelvic dysfunction**.

My research documented a pudendal nerve trial which consisted of 25 patients who presented with pudendal nerve pain. The patients had been referred by doctors on the suspicion that their issues were musculoskeletal related. The research revealed Level B2 evidence that treating sacroiliac dysfunction gave a success rate of 95 per cent in treating their symptoms.

Therefore, in the following chapters, I will explain how certain patients who have a diagnosis of Pudendal Neuropathy or its subheadings, pudendal neuralgia and PNE, may be managed as a musculoskeletal condition, particularly as it relates to pelvic dysfunction.

Consequently, as an initial priority, for these pelvic pain patients, I believe an efficient differential diagnosis should concentrate on assessing the possibility of lumbar-pelvic and sacroiliac joint dysfunction. Generally, this can be accomplished simply in the clinical setting by a skilled physiotherapist or musculoskeletal health professional. The only external investigation may include a specialised MRN to determine the possibility of the presence of real entrapment, but this, from my experience, probably is rare. As well, I would deliver a warning that an MRN 'positive' result can be definitely misleading regarding directing the choice of treatment. Even though it may show entrapment, or scarring, a musculoskeletal approach can often adequately 'release' the nerve and treat the condition.

Ultimately, if you find no indication that pelvic dysfunction is involved, you must, of course, continue to consider other possibilities, most of which have already been mentioned. A word here on surgery. This should only be considered after every conservative method of treatment has been exhausted. For various reasons, a certain small percentage of cases will have such rigid nerve impingement or entrapment that surgical intervention may be the only reasonable way to go.

Summary

What should be clear by now is the complex nature of CPPS. According to a study by Weiss[5], it is no wonder that for these patients, the mean time to the diagnosis of pudendal neuropathy (pudendal neuralgia or PNE) is about four years; they have seen 10–30 Health Professionals; have suffered innumerable invasive and non-invasive procedures; have developed significant central and peripheral sensitization with the concomitant allodynia and hyperalgesia; have developed an attitude of hopelessness and have become markedly depressed to the point of committing suicide.

It can be realised that any compromise in the nerves ability to work efficiently and effectively can potentially have serious and drastic effects. These effects are not only physical, setting up situations of chronic pain and inherently interfering with sexual, urological and gastric functions, they can be psychological, social and emotional, impacting significantly on self-worth, identity and relationships. Misdiagnosed, unaddressed or inadequately treated, pelvic pain syndromes involving the pudendal nerve and other pelvic nerves can very clearly then contribute to unsound mental health, and can prospectively spiral a patient into reactive depression and anxiety.

In the following chapter I will take you through the anatomy, musculoskeletal assessment and the treatment, followed by a discussion on continued management and prevention.

So you've got pelvic pain ... Here's how to manage it.

Anatomy, Biomechanics and Pathology

The three main anatomical structures we need to understand, particularly in relation to pelvic pain, are the pelvic girdle, the sacroiliac joint and the pudendal nerve. However, other nerves and joints are often associated with, and can also contribute to, the phenomenon of pelvic pain, so I will identify and examine their roles as well.

The Pelvic Girdle

The pelvis is a bony ring at the base of the vertebral column, or spine. It is comprised of four bones, the *sacrum* and the *coccyx,* which are an extension of the spine, and the two *innominate* bones (or nameless bones), which flank either side of the sacrum. The upper section of the innominate bone is called the *ilium* (*ilia* means flank), and it attaches to the sacrum at the sacroiliac joint (SIJ). (See Figure 1)

Stability is achieved by maintaining compression across the ring, and is dependant on deep interosseous and long dorsal ligaments posterior to the SIJs.

The Sacroiliac Joint

The SIJ is a synovial joint and is the largest and strongest joint of the body. It provides a dynamic and mobile link between the vertebral column and the

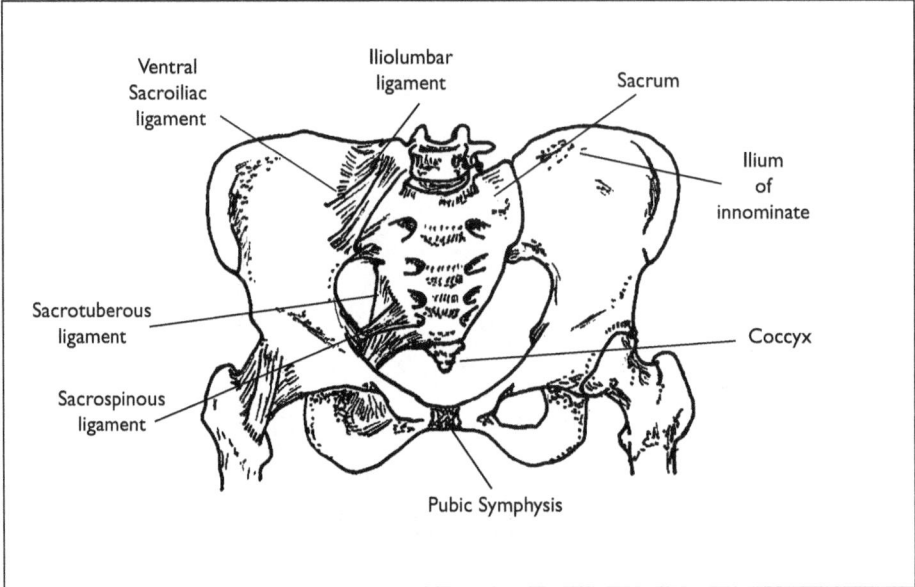

Figure 1. The Pelvis and the Sacroiliac Joint (front view)

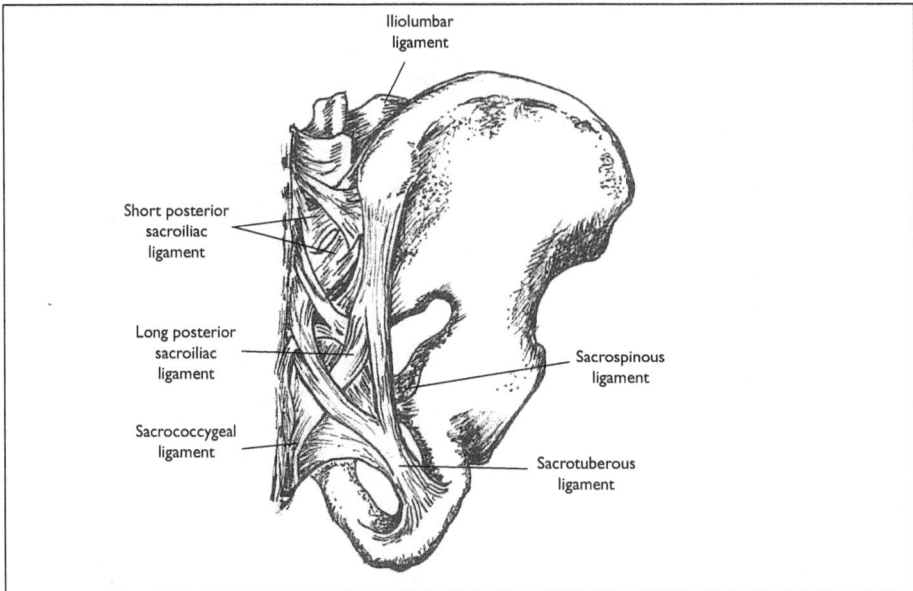

Figure 2. The Pelvis and the Sacroiliac Joint (back view)

lower limb, distributing weight down the spine through the SIJ and down the leg. (See Figures 1 and 2)

The joint basically functions as a shock absorber, being lined with tough hyaline and fibrous cartilage. It is also supported by a blending of powerful ligaments and articular capsule. The articular surface is L-shaped, developing a variety of irregular elevations and depressions. These configurations produce an interlocking of the two bones that assist in creating great stability.

Of clinical interest, particularly in relation to treatment procedures using mobilising techniques, is that the joint exhibits at least two planes of movement, often three, slightly angulated to one another.

However, while SIJ mobility has been shown to be limited, significant movement does occur (Lee, 2011)[1]. Several studies agree that the average rotation of the innominate bone on the sacrum in the weight-bearing position is probably less than 2.5 degrees with about 1 mm of translation. The research suggests if the joint rotates more than 6 degrees and translates more than 2 mm, pathologic changes (damage or trauma) would most probably occur. (Jacob & Kissling, 1995)[2]

It is this mechanism that I propose may compromise the pudendal nerve. The putative reasoning suggests that if extreme physical stress causes the ilium to excessively rotate on the sacrum or the sacrum to rotate excessively on the ilium, (potentially damaging the SIJ), compression may be placed on the pudendal nerve as it moves and stretches between various pelvic anatomical structures. Most researchers and clinicians suggest that this may occur, in particular, between the sacrospinous and sacrotuberous ligaments, as well as in the Alcock's canal. The sacrospinous and sacrotuberous ligaments attach the sacrum to the innominate bones below the SIJ and are considered to be accessory ligaments. [Detachment of these ligaments (by surgery) apparently does not affect stability.]

It is suggested that as a result of excessive innominate bone or sacral rotation, significant soft tissue damage occurs to the SIJ ligaments, over and above any neural involvement. As these ligaments heal, fibrotic scar tissue forms, the joint may stiffen (in a malaligned position) and ostensibly can result in chronic SIJ restrictions. This change in the pelvic girdle biomechanics may then exert unremitting pressure on the pudendal nerve, giving rise to serious neural symptoms, including pain and sensitisation. Assessment is aimed at revealing the particular restriction of motion where the joint is 'stuck'. (see Chapter 2) The treatment is to restore that motion.

The Pudendal Nerve

The pudendal nerve gains its name from the Latin word '*pudenda*', which means 'private parts,' or 'the shamefuls'. It is a mixed nerve containing somatic fibres (sensory and motor) and autonomic fibres. The autonomic fibres constitute that part of the visceral nervous system that functions automatically, affecting micturition, perspiration, sexual arousal, skin changes, etc. This means the pudendal nerve has the facility to transfer messages (hot, cold, etc.) to the central nervous system. It can also transfer messages, both to control active movements (in particular to some of the pelvic floor muscles, including the bladder and bowel sphincters), as well as to control involuntary bodily functions, such as erectile ability and bladder and bowel functions. In fact, the pudendal nerve is a major contributor to bladder control. Essentially, the pudendal nerve is mainly involved with what the ancients deemed as shameful — the sexual organs. (Figures 3a, b, c, d).

The pudendal nerve emerges from the sacral plexus, gaining fibres primarily from the second, third, and fourth anterior sacral nerve roots (S2, S3, and S4) and (autonomic) sympathetic fibres from the lower sympathetic chain. It does receive other contributions from S1 and S5. This is an important point, particularly considering the role of S1 and its connections to the lumbar and sacral nerves (See Figures 3a, b). It is therefore possible for some patients with sciatic nerve symptoms, regardless of the cause, to have symptoms referred into the pudendal nerve.

As several of the **lumbar** nerves, in particular, the inferior gluteal nerve, the tibial (medial popliteal) nerve, the common peroneal (lateral popliteal) nerve, and the perforating cutaneous nerve, and the **sacral** nerve, (posterior femoral cutaneous nerve), derive at least one connection from S2, S3, or S4, the patient may also complain of pain in the lower back, groin, buttock, posterior thigh, calf or foot.

This pain may be referred either by neural convergence, direct injury to the lumbar area, or chronic SIJ damage impacting on L5, S1, thereby interfering with local emitting lumbar and sacral nerves. Given the wide range of innervation of the SIJ and its adjacent neural structures, SIJ capsular stimulation may also refer various pain patterns to the groin, buttock, thigh, calf or foot.

The pudendal nerve follows a tortuous course outside and through the pelvis. As such, it exits the pelvic cavity approximately 3 cm below the SIJ, under the piriformis muscle, a site that researchers speculate can entrap the nerve. It then moves through the greater sciatic foramen, and descends on the underside of the sacrotuberous ligament.

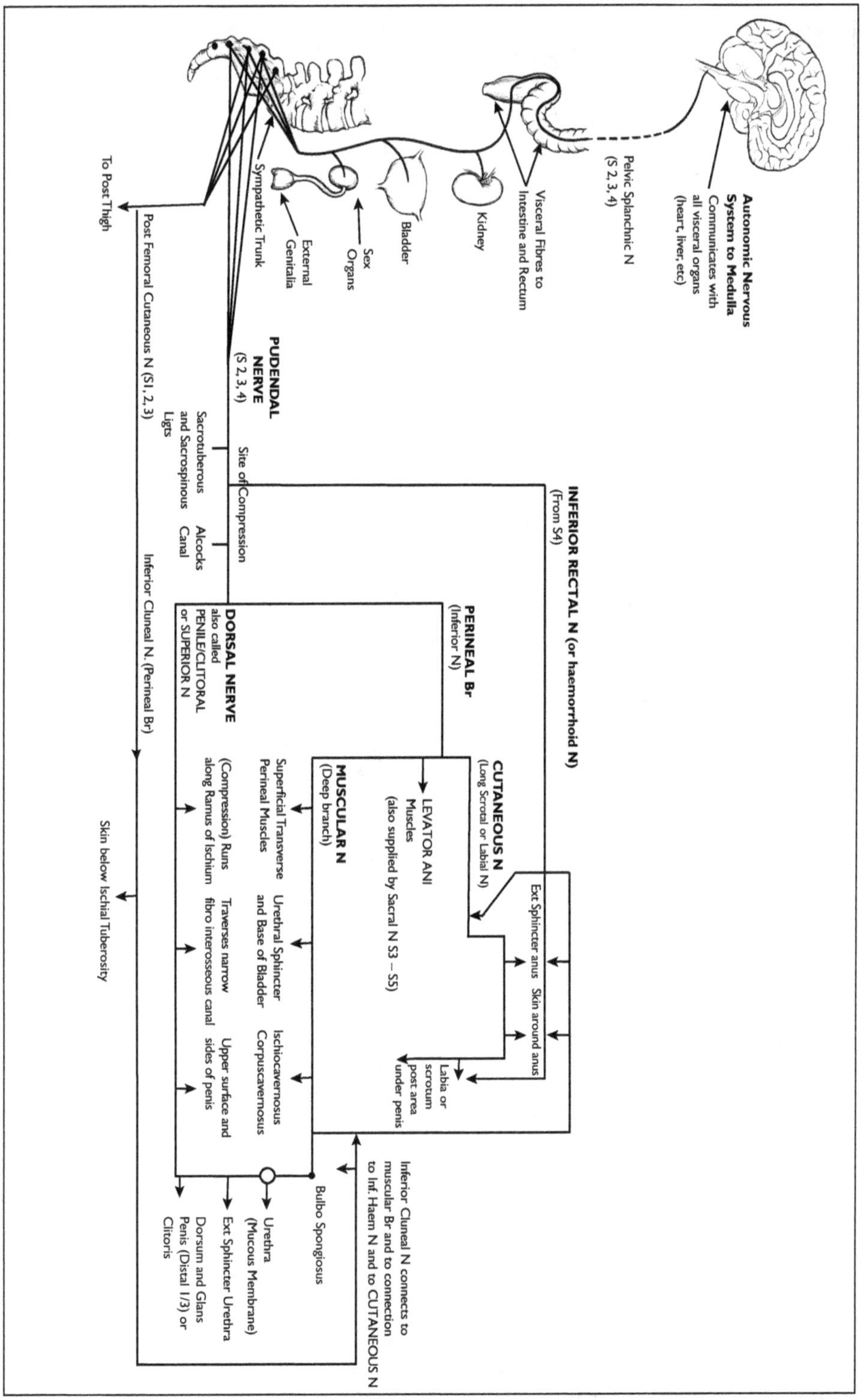

Figure 3a Pudendal Nerve Map

MUSCULAR NERVE (DEEP BRANCH OF PERINEAL NERVE).

Perineal muscles, Levator Ani, Urethral External Sphincter and Base of Bladder, muscles of arousal/erectile ability and ejaculation

to

Can lead to:
- Pain after micturition
- Voiding Problems
- Slow stream
- Pelvic floor pain and spasm
- Low abdominal pain
- Erectile Dysfunction
- Priapism
- Persistent Arousal
- Pain after ejaculation
- Pain during sex
- Urinary urgency
- Urinary frequency

DORSAL NERVE OF PENIS (or Clitoris)

Will give pain and numbness to penis, clitoris.

CUTANEOUS BRANCH OF PERINEAL NERVE (Scrotal N.) or (Labial N.)

to

Scrotum or Labia, will give:
- Pain in scrotum, labia and area under penis
- Redness, itchiness scrotum
- Testicle feels drawn into pelvis

INFERIOR RECTAL NERVE S4 to

External sphincter and skin around anus. Can lead to:
- Pain after defaecation
- Faecal Urgency
- Irritable bowel syndromes
- Altered sensations in bowel
- Knife or lump in anus

Labels:
- PELVIC BONE (Innominate)
- SACROILIAC JOINT
- BLADDER
- EXTERNAL URINARY SPHINCTER (Part of Lev. Ani)
- PROSTATE
- LEVATOR ANI
- PUDENDAL CANAL (Alcocks)
- SACRUM
- SACRAL PLEXUS
- PUDENDAL NERVE
- OBTURATOR INTERNUS
- SACROSPINOUS LIGAMENT
- COCCYX
- SACROTUBEROUS LIGAMENT
- PERINEAL NERVE
- FALCIFORM PROCESS OF SACROTUBEROUS LIGAMENT

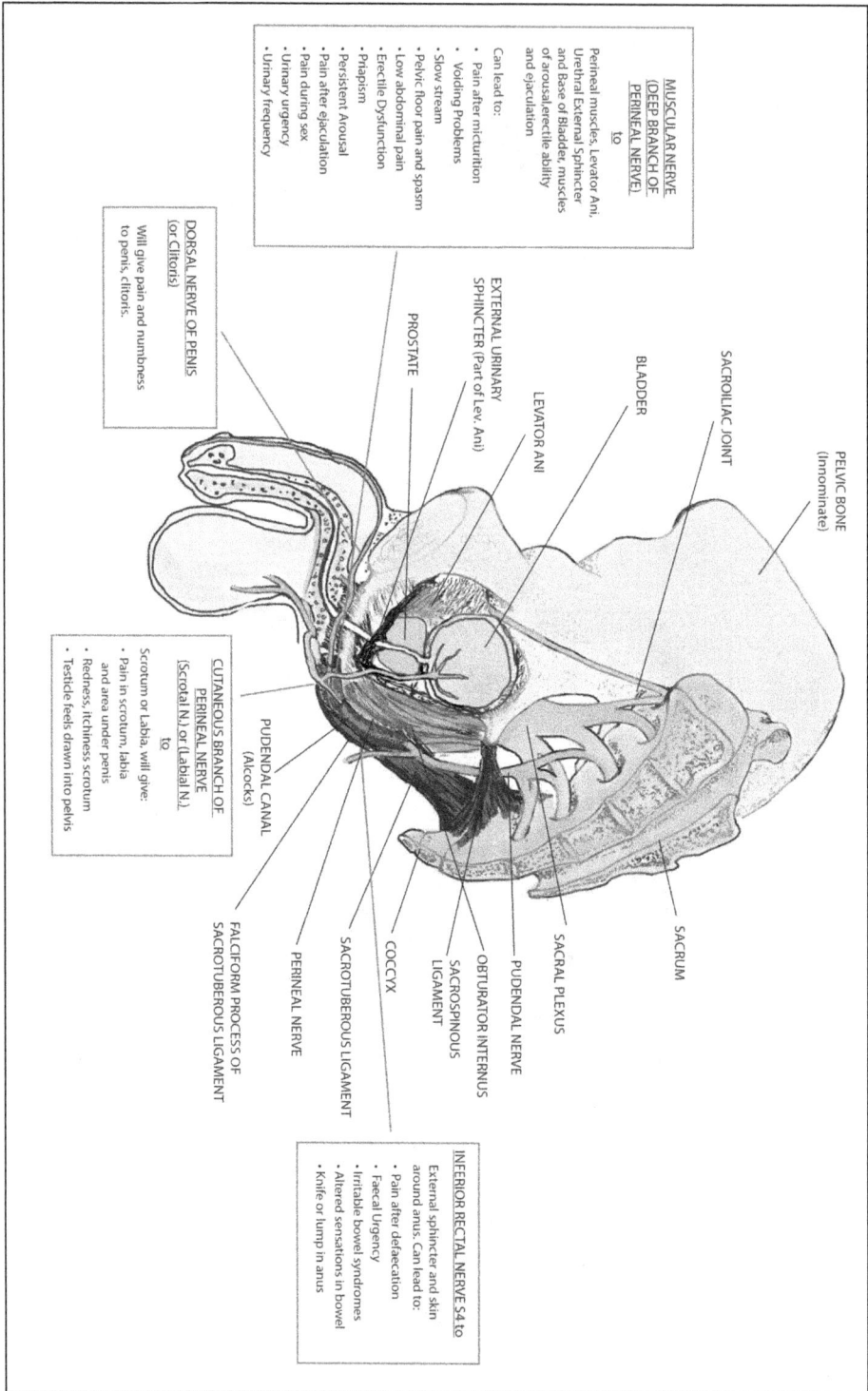

Figure 3b. Pudendal Nerve — Distribution and Functions

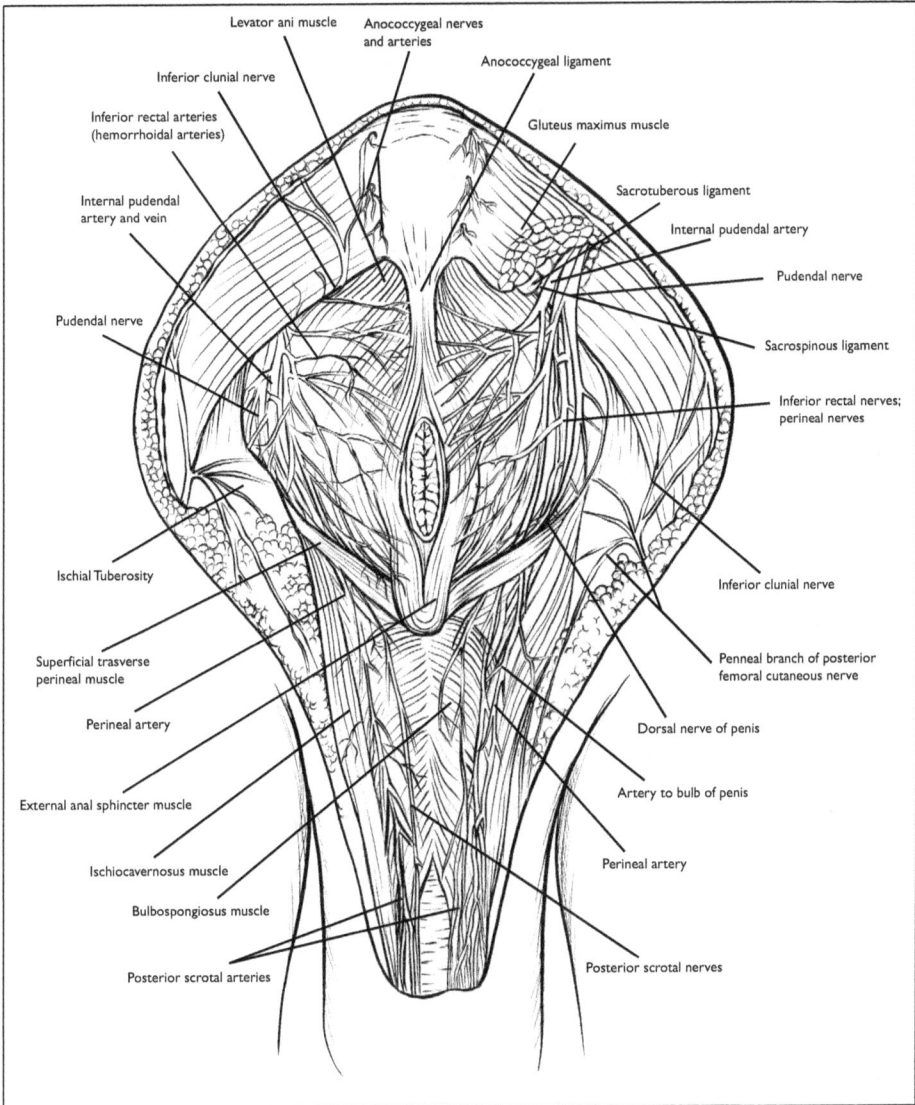

Figure 3c. The Male Pudendal Nerve

At this point, the nerve then divides into three main terminal branches — the inferior rectal nerve, the perineal nerve and the dorsal nerve of the penis (or clitoris).

Early on, the inferior rectal nerve (or haemorrhoid nerve) leaves the pudendal nerve. In fact, recent research suggests 40% of the rectal nerve originates directly from S4 root, and 60% travels with the pudendal nerve. The nerve makes its way to supply the anal sphincter and the skin around the anus, particularly below the ischial tuberosity (connecting with the inferior cluneal nerve). The

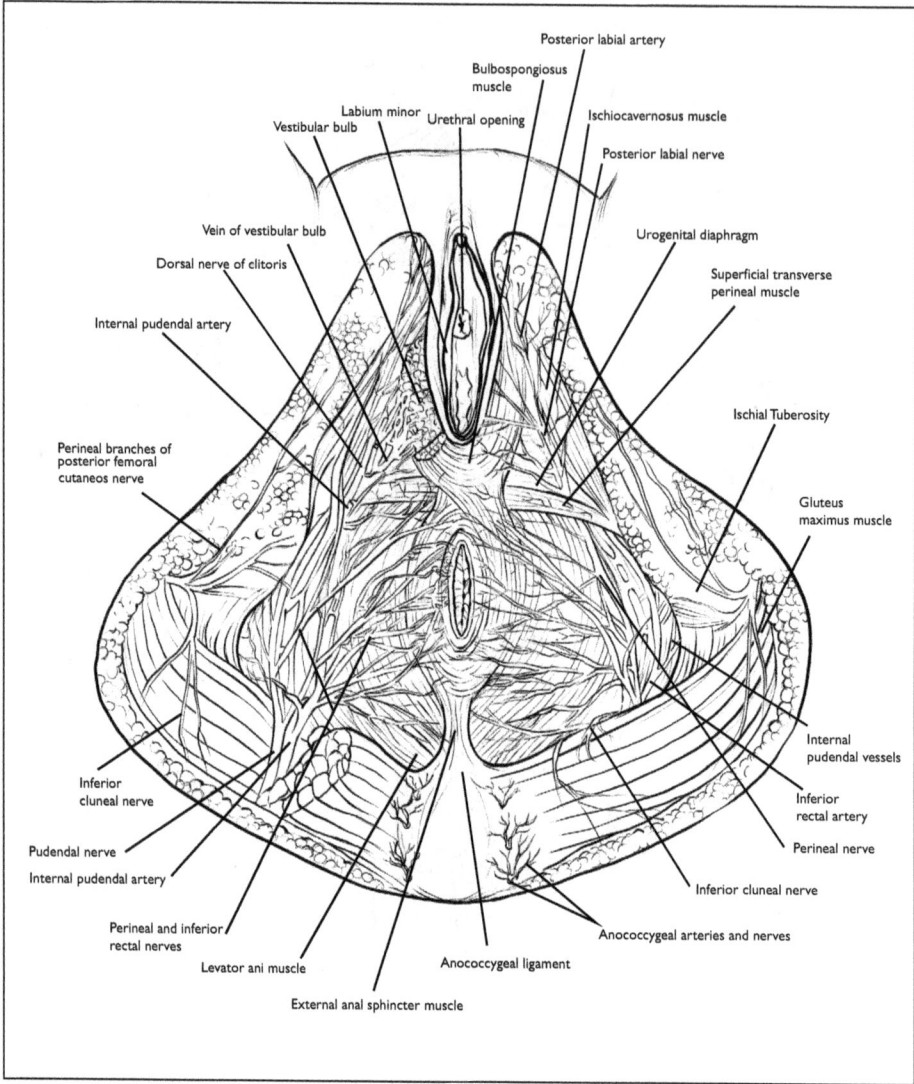

Figure 3d. The Female Pudendal Nerve

pudendal nerve then passes under the sacrospinous ligament on the inside of the ischial spine and re-enters the pelvic cavity through the lesser sciatic foramen immediately adjacent to the sacrospinous ligament.

This is the area where most researchers and clinicians speculate that the nerve has a high probable chance of being 'entrapped' between the sacrospinous and sacrotuberous ligaments. Researchers also consider the nerve can be trapped by the falciform process of the sacrotuberous ligament (the broad attachment of the sacrotuberous ligament on the ischial tuberosity).

Once the nerve has re-entered the pelvis, it travels upwards and forwards along the wall of the ischiorectal fossa underneath the obturator fascia. This is another area, the obturator fascia in the Alcock's canal within the obturator internus muscle, where it is speculated the nerve may become pinched and cause irritation.

Neurodynamic testing can be applied here. As the obturator internus is an external rotator of the thigh, placing the leg in internal rotation may increase symptoms as the muscle and the nerve become stretched. Functionally, many patients with pudendal neuralgia cannot perform a deep squat or split squat without pain in some or all of the pudendal nerve distribution, particularly if there is suspicion the nerve may be irritated as it moves between the sacrospinous and sacrotuberous ligaments or the Alcock's canal.

Here, the pudendal nerve divides into the other two terminal branches — the **perineal** (also called the **inferior** branch), and the **dorsal** nerve of the penis/clitoris, (also called the **superior** nerve). Researchers have noted where these two nerves leave the main trunk after the Alcock's canal, they do so at an angle. As mentioned earlier, they also speculate that this may increase the chances of compression and/or entrapment.

The dorsal (or penile/clitoral) nerve can be endangered in this area as it runs along the ramus of the ischium (the part of the pelvis you sit on while riding a bike) towards the pubic symphysis. (It can be easily compressed here by sitting on a poor-fitting bicycle seat, resulting in penile numbness/pain.) In the female, a painful allodynia response can be elicited by entering the vagina and palpating the nerve along the ischial ramus.

Further, the dorsal nerve can be endangered as it approaches the pubic symphysis in an area where it traverses a narrow fibro-osseous canal. Researchers speculate this area may also increase the risk of compression and/or entrapment. The nerve then supplies the upper surface and sides of the penis and the dorsum and distal third of the glans (or the clitoris). It also sends a connection, with the sympathetic nerves from the pelvic plexus (the cavernous nerve), to the muscular nerve (or deep branch) and the corpus cavernosum muscle.

Of interest, this is the same connection, with the cavernous nerve, which can lead to erectile dysfunction during prostate surgery (radical prostatectomy). It is part of the large neurovascular plexus that surrounds the prostate. The cavernous nerves arise from cells behind the prostate from the preganglionic pelvic splanchnic nerves (S2, S3, S4).

In the meantime, the perineal branch (or the inferior nerve) actually divides into two branches, forming the **cutaneous** branch, (or **long scrotal nerve** or **labial nerve)**, and the deep **muscular** branch.

The muscular branch follows along to innervate the Levator ani muscle (which lifts the pelvic floor), most of the muscles that supply the perineum (the area between the scrotum and the anus), the urethral sphincter and base of the bladder and the muscles that allow erectile function (for penis and clitoris). Irritation of this nerve can lead to erectile dysfunction and pain on ejaculation (for males), and pain on arousal and/or orgasm (in females). It can also lead to urinary urgency and frequency and pain in the bladder and supra pubic region, as well as inefficient (incomplete or slow) voiding. However, because the bladder is also controlled by a complex system involving the hypogastric nerve (T11, T12, L1, L2), this tie-up must be considered when investigating urinary function causes. These joints (T11, T12, L1, L2) must be assessed as well as S2, S3, S4 (the SIJ). (See Figure 4.)

It is useful to understand a little more of how the bladder works.

The Internal Urethral Sphincter Nerves

The nerves that control the urethral sphincter can be described as follows:

- Parasympathetic nerves from the S2, S3 and S4 levels of the spinal cord control the internal sphincter, causing it to relax to allow urine to pass out of the bladder.

- Sympathetic nerves from the T11 to L2 levels of the spinal cord cause the internal urethral sphincter to tighten, helping to hold stored urine in the bladder.

- Both of these functions are involuntary. This means that they operate in an automatic or reflex way, beyond one's control.

The External Urethral Sphincter Nerves

- Nerves from the pudendal nerve, muscular branch, S2–S4 levels of the spinal cord control the external urethral sphincter. This sphincter is able to be voluntarily or consciously controlled (see Figure 4).

Filling and Emptying the Bladder

When the amount of urine in the bladder reaches around 250 ml, sensors in the bladder muscle are stimulated. The bladder signals the brain, and one will feel a slight urge to pass urine. Once one has around 400–500 ml in the bladder, this urge grows in intensity and one needs to empty his or her bladder.

When full, the stretch receptors in the bladder stimulate nerves to initiate the subconscious reflex called the micturition reflex. The final stage of urination

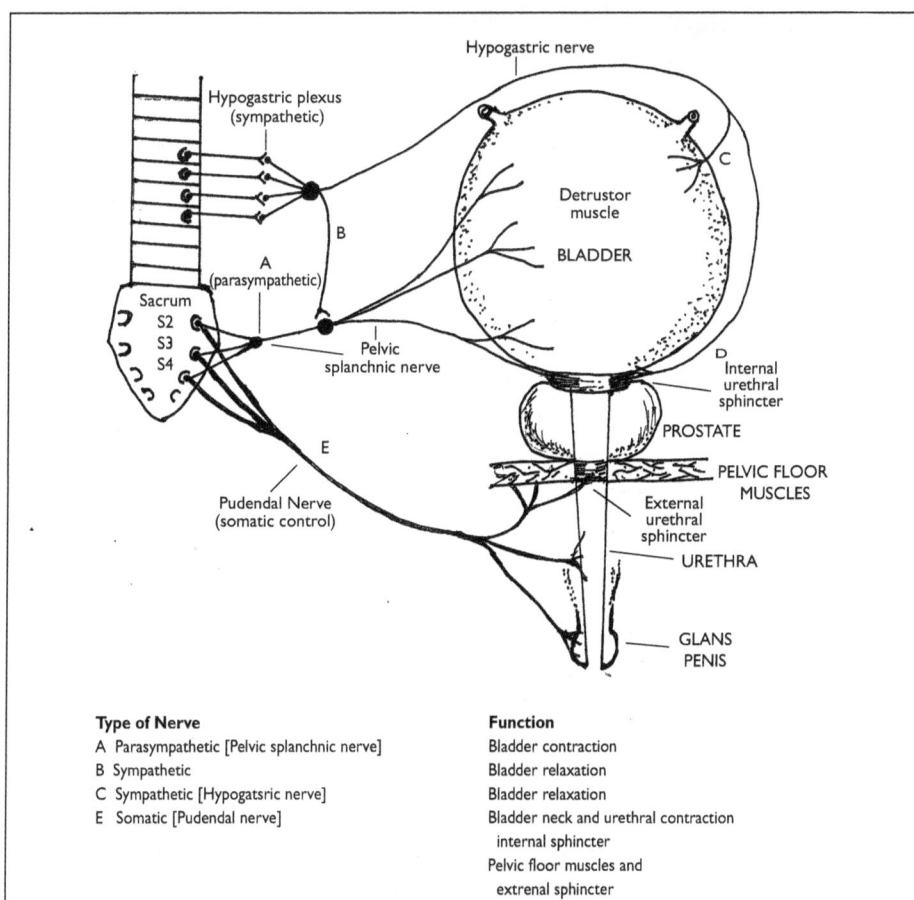

Type of Nerve	Function
A Parasympathetic [Pelvic splanchnic nerve]	Bladder contraction
B Sympathetic	Bladder relaxation
C Sympathetic [Hypogatsric nerve]	Bladder relaxation
E Somatic [Pudendal nerve]	Bladder neck and urethral contraction
	internal sphincter
	Pelvic floor muscles and
	extrenal sphincter

Figure 4. Nerve Supply to Bladder

remains in one's conscious control, until one can access an appropriate place to void and relax the external sphincter.

Urinary Urgency

Urge incontinence is described as an inability to defer urination, usually accompanied by a strong urge or 'need to go'. Patients simply can't 'hold on'.

Urge incontinence occurs when the circuitry to the brain becomes confused. There are many known causes, mainly relating to the bladder wall muscle (detrusor muscle), hypogastric nerve (T11, T12, L1, L2), the pelvic floor muscles and external urinary sphincter (S2, S3, S4) reacting to any number of inappropriate stimuli and over-contracting, setting off the sensation of needing to 'go'. Such causes can be bladder stones, urinary tract infections, neurological conditions, enlarged prostate, anxiety reactions and conditioned responses (putting the key in the front door, running water).

Whatever the cause, most cases of urge incontinence develop because the bladder and pelvic floor muscles have taken over command of the urinary process. This reflex circuitry imbalance can also be caused by compromise of either the pudendal nerve or the hypogastric nerve (or both). Therefore, it is important to assess both these nerves at their spinal origins, particularly looking for sacroiliac joint dysfunction in relation to the potential for it to impact on the pudendal nerve.

There may be a need here to complement the treatment program by strengthening the pelvic floor muscles with the aim of overriding the flawed messages going to the bladder telling it to void early. There may be a case here also to introduce the concept of 'bladder training', learning how to resist the sensation of urgency and postpone the voiding. Distracting thoughts, watching television, reading, etc., can also be helpful in diverting attention from the urge.

Nerve Supplies to Anal Sphincter and the Rectum

The muscular branch of the pudendal nerve also sends a slip to the **inferior rectal nerve** (Figures 3a, b) and one to the **inferior cluneal nerve** (or perineal branch of the posterior femoral cutaneous nerve), which supplies the skin below the ischial tuberosity (see Figure 5).

The long scrotal/labial nerve (or cutaneous) branch curves below and to the back of the ischiorectal fossa, pierces the fascia lata, and runs to the skin behind the scrotum and in the area under the shaft of the penis in males and the external labia in females. Along the way the nerve innervates the anus and the sphincter ani (the muscles that control the anus). The nerve also communicates with the inferior rectal (haemorrhoidal) nerve which, as mentioned previously, leaves the pudendal nerve very early on. This nerve supplies the skin around the anus and also the external sphincter ani. The actual rectum is supplied by L1, L2 and parasympathetic fibres of S2, S3, S4.
The external anal sphincter lies in contact with and surrounds the internal anal sphincter. The muscles have different nerve supplies and different functions.

The external anal sphincter is a voluntary sphincter innervated primarily by the inferior rectal nerve of the pudendal nerve, mainly S4. This enables an individual to consciously squeeze (close) the external anal sphincter. This nerve also carries sensory input from the lower anal canal and the skin around the anus. It is therefore sensitive to pain, temperature and touch. Interestingly, the motor supply to the external anal sphincter is carried bilaterally by the pudendal nerve.

The internal anal sphincter is an involuntary muscle supplied by the parasympathetic fibres, mainly originating from the hypogastric plexus, T10, T11, T12, L1, L2, and passes along the pelvic splanchnic nerves. Its work is done automatically, so we have no conscious control of it. The organ and nerve only registers stretch, not pain.

Clinically, this is important as patients who complain of pain during and after defecation (and no pain at the beginning of defecation) should be assessed for external anal sphincter nerve supply compromise — check S4 (by palpation).

While the majority of the pelvic floor muscles are innervated by the pudendal nerve, several workers have shown that puborectalis is innervated below by the pudendal nerve (inferior rectal) and from above by the sacral nerves. It has been found that pudendal nerve damage may cause dysfunction of the puborectalis and may cause faecal incontinence.

A point to remember – All of these nerves and their connections, as well as the associated ligaments, have been found to have many variations. The discussion in this book therefore is a useful generality. In fact, at the Nice (France) Pelvic Pain Conference 2015, Professor Roger Robert of Nantes stated that anatomical variations are always a problem for surgery, particularly at the Alcock's canal.

Other Nerves, Including Thoracolumbar, Lumbar and Sacral Nerves

To reinforce the complexities involved when dealing with the pelvic neural system, several communicating lumbar nerves (from L1 and L2), the iliohypogastric, ilioinguinal and genital branch of the genitofemoral, also send branches to the scrotum (or upper vulva and labia majora) (see Figure 7). The anatomy of these three nerves is extremely variable and they can also send branches to the skin of the lower abdomen, groin and pubic area, and to the upper and inner parts of the thigh. Pain in this area is often misdiagnosed as groin, adductor muscle tendonitis, 'sports hernia' or pubic symphysis (osteitis pubis involvement). Femoroacetabular joint degeneration and labial tear can also be a cause of recalcitrant groin pain. The genitofemoral nerve also supplies the cremaster muscle, a not-so-common area presenting as a painful symptom.

Trauma to the femoral branch of the genitofemoral nerve causes hypoesthesia (numbness) over the anterior thigh below the inguinal ligament, distinguishing the nerve from iliohypogastric and ilioinguinal nerves. [Note that pain (or numbness) from these nerves can occur immediately following an abdominal surgery.]

Further, the prostate and the upper part of the bladder receives its nerve supply from this same iliohypogastric plexus, while the base and neck of the bladder predominately receives its supply from the sacral plexus, including the pudendal nerve.

Another lumbar nerve, the obturator (from L2, L3 and L4), can also refer pain via cutaneous sensory branches to the outer layers of the inner thigh, the hip and medial knee. The anterior branch of this nerve innervates the main adductor muscles of the thigh, the adductor longus, adductor brevis and gracilis muscle. The posterior branch innervates the obturator externus, portions of the adductor magnus and the pectineus muscle. (See Figures 7a and b.) Symptoms from these areas are often diagnosed as obturator nerve entrapment, and relief has been obtained by surgery to release scarring at the level of the obturator foramen. It is essential therefore, to examine L2, L3 and L4 for potential dysfunction to consider mobilising as a treatment.

A word here on chronic irritable bowel syndrome (IBS). It is worthwhile considering the potential of the pudendal nerve (particularly S4) as a cause for bowel pain, so it is important to explore sacroiliac joint dysfunction. Otherwise, as with any chronic pain syndrome, there will be issues in the nerves themselves, in the brain and the brain's coping mechanism.

The largest lumbar nerve, the femoral nerve (from L3 and L4) supplies the iliacus, pectineus and the muscles on the front of the thigh, with cutaneous filaments going to the front and inner side of the thigh and to the leg and the foot. It also supplies articular branches to the front of the knee. Compromise of this nerve can also produce symptoms in the buttock, front of the thigh and knee.

Another important area to consider relates to the thoracolumbar region. The tenth thoracic nerve, where it leaves through the fourth sacral segment, innervate the reproductive organs, abdominal wall, low back, thighs and the pelvic floor. The twelfth thoracic to the fourth lumbar segments can refer pain to the lower abdomen, iliopsoas, quadratus lumborum, piriformis and obturator internus muscles.

Along these lines, one explanation for some of the symptoms is that they may be caused by a dysfunction in the thoracolumbar junction as described by Dr. Robert Maigne[3, 4]. Maigne stated that referred pain from spinal nerves T12 and L1 can manifest itself as lower back pain that mimics pain of lumbosacral or sacroiliac origin. It is thought some of this pain is mediated via the superior cluneal nerves (L1, L2, L3). Referred pain from spinal nerves originating from here can also be felt in the lower abdomen, the medial aspect of the upper thigh and the groin, labia majora or scrotum.

Searching for stiffness and/or pain by passive movements and palpation of the T12, L1 joint is the most effective assessment method. Treatment in this case includes spinal manipulation of the thoracolumbar region, and Maigne suggests, infiltration of the painful zygapophysial joint with a corticosteroid. (see Figure 7c, Maigne's Syndrome)

To complete the review, another subgroup of patients report pain in sitting, which is relieved by standing and peculiarly, by sitting on a toilet seat. This is generally caused by pressure being applied to a branch of the posterior femoral cutaneous nerve (or posterior cutaneous nerve of the thigh). The posterior femoral cutaneous nerve itself arises from S1, S2, and S3 and provides innervations to the skin of the posterior surface of the thigh and leg, as well as to the skin of the lateral perineum, labia majora and clitoris. The particular branch, the perineal branch (or inferior cluneal nerve), swings medially below the ischial tuberosity and refers pain to the upper and medial side of the gluteal muscle and thigh and to the perineum. Thus, while sitting on a toilet seat, there will be much reduced or no pressure on this nerve as the pressure is applied laterally (off the sensitive area).

As with the pudendal nerve, Darnis and colleagues[5] have documented that the inferior cluneal nerve can be compressed at the level of the sacrotuberous ligament and can also be compromised along its passage under the ischium. J.J. Labat (Toulouse Pelvic Pain Conference 2015) advises that hydrocortisone injection makes no difference to the outcome.

The management here initially is to look for a SIJ dysfunction. This is in case the posterior cutaneous nerve of the thigh is compromised at its origin, S1, S2 and S3. Begin by mobilising the SIJ (as per 'Treatment' in Chapter 3), then aim to desensitise the nerves by reducing pressure on them while sitting. Always sit on a 'modified' type of seat (a personalised cushion with the centre and front section removed), or simply stand if possible. If that doesn't settle the symptoms, arrange for a magnetic resonance neurography (MRN) of the inferior cluneal nerve to test for local damage (or entrapment) here — a rare occurrence, I might add.

The other nerves to consider are the superior cluneal (L1, L2, L3), which innervate the skin of the upper and lateral part of the buttocks, and the middle cluneal nerves (S1, S2, S3), which supply the middle area of the buttocks (see Figures 6 and 7). Clinicians have noticed that these cluneal nerves can be restricted in their osteofibrous tunnels. Once again, assess by palpating the appropriate joints, searching for stiffness/pain. The initial conservative treatment should be to mobilise the appropriate joints L1, L2, L3, or S1, S2, and S3. Active surgical release is a common treatment for all three cluneal nerves.

Of interest to men who suffer scrotal pain (and this is 80% of men whom I see with pudendal neuralgia), and women who have labia or vulva pain, the long scrotal nerve (labial nerve for females) is probably the main offending

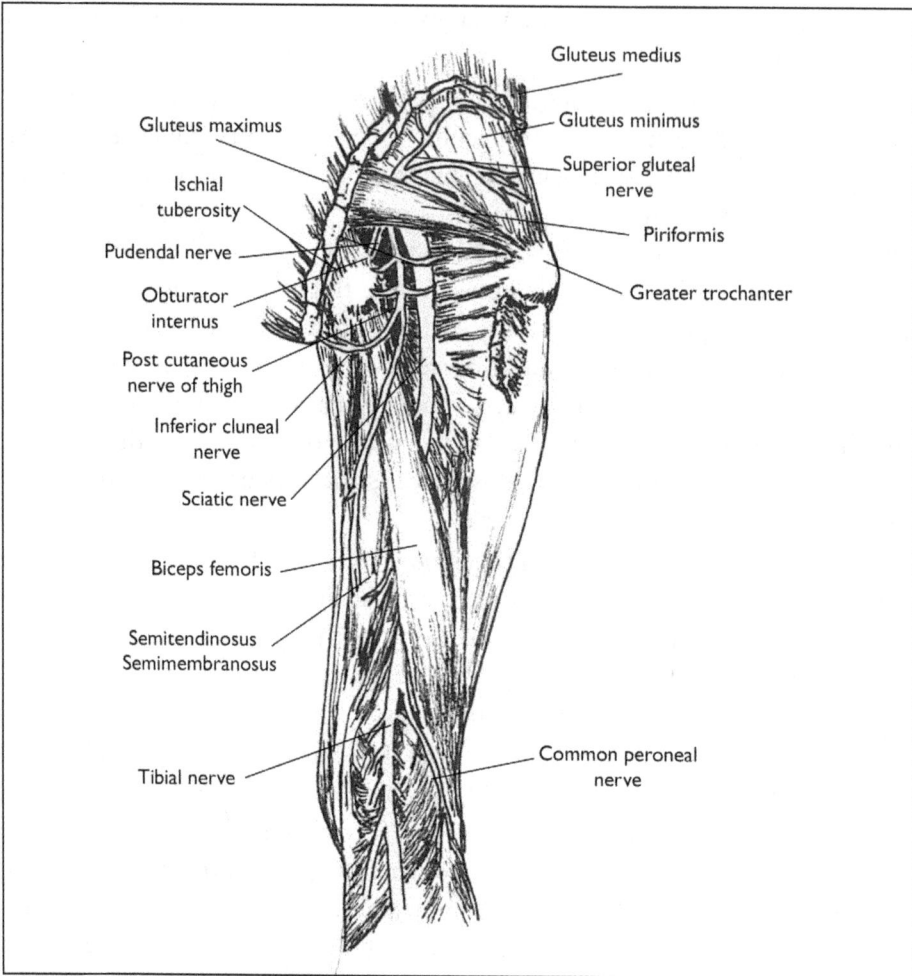

Figure 5. Inferior Cluneal Nerve (or Perineal Branch of Posterior Femoral Cutaneous Nerve)

culprit. However, the difficulty in diagnosing the origin of scrotal pain (or labia pain) is clearly obvious. As has been detailed previously, many nerves actually communicate with the scrotum (or labia):

- Long scrotal nerve (or labial nerve) of the pudendal nerve (S2, S3, S4)
- Lumbar nerves (iliohypogastric, ilioinguinal and genitofemoral — L1, L2)
- Thoroco-lumbar junction, T12, L1 (Maigne's Syndrome)
- Posterior-femoral cutaneous nerve (S1, S2, S3) via the inferior cluneal nerve

Regardless, an investigation into the possibility of pelvic dysfunction, lumbar spinal involvement or Maigne's Syndrome will generally address most of these

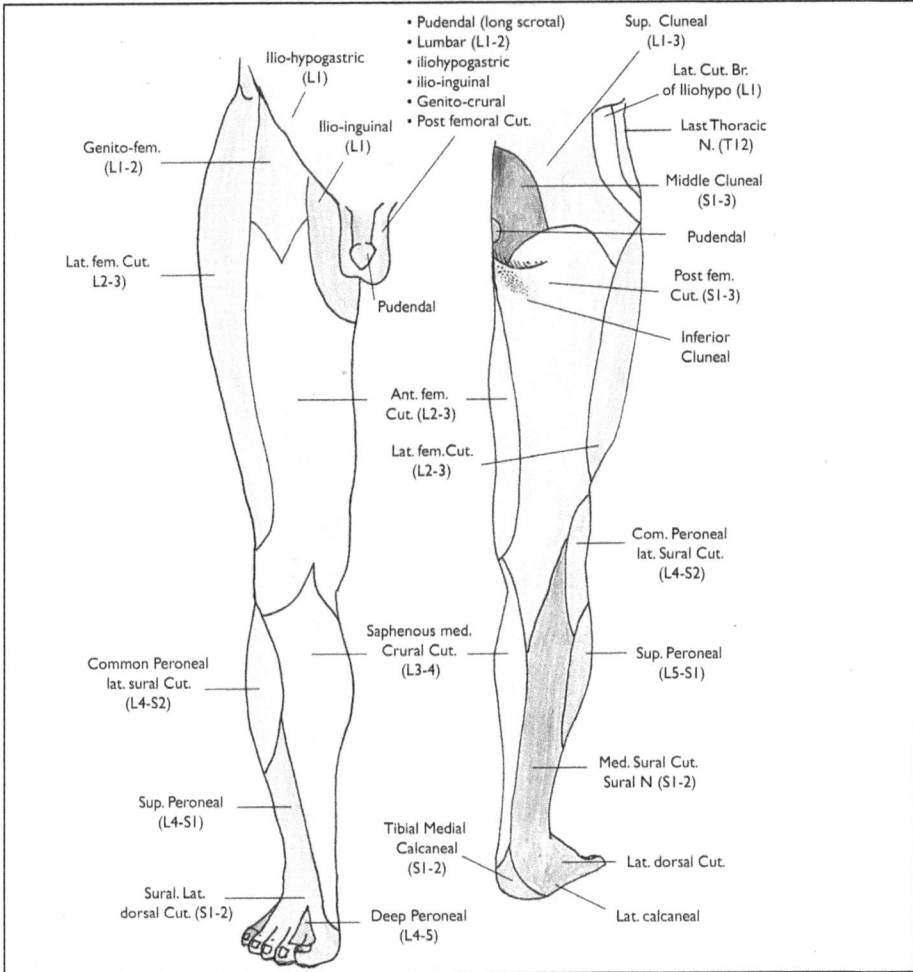

Figure 6. Cutaneous Nerves of the Lower limb (Pain particularly in the scrotal skin)

cases. (**Note:** The testes (and ovary), epididymis and vas deferens are innervated by thoracolumbar nerve roots T10–T11, not the pudendal nerve.)

A Discussion on Pain after Orgasm and Ejaculation

Ejaculatory and orgasmic pain is a common complaint in men with chronic pelvic pain syndrome (CPPS). The cause of this is controversial, but some studies have shown it can impact on 75% of men with CPPS in the first three months. As could be expected, the negative impact on individuals increased with the frequency of their ejaculatory pain, and their mental and physical quality of life decreased. Some researchers have suggested neuromuscular spasm of the pelvic

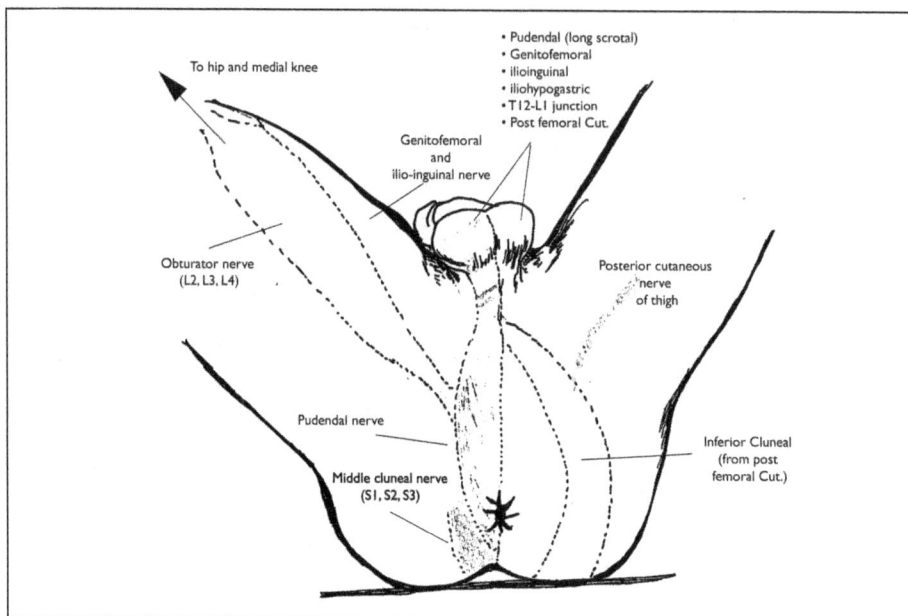

Figure 7a. Innervation of the Perineum

floor muscles may represent an important source of this ejaculatory pain — either as a primary or secondary central nervous system disturbance in regulation of the pelvic floor muscles. Tension myalgia associated with abnormally high pelvic floor muscle tone can therefore be a significant component of pain and dysfunction in men with CPPS.

Neuromuscular re-education has been shown to result in reduced baseline tone of the pelvic floor muscles. When applied appropriately, various manual techniques can be employed by certified and experienced pelvic floor physiotherapists to address this painful dysfunction. Mindfulness and targeted paradoxical relaxation training for tense muscle groups (pelvic floor, abdominal and adductor muscle groups) have also been helpful. This involves first performing a volitional contraction then deliberately relaxing the muscles.

Along these lines, I also find it useful to suggest to the male patient that during orgasm, he should not try to heighten the climax by actively using his pelvic floor muscles. He should allow the action to be a more natural and relaxed event, such as steady and dome shaped, not a sudden high-peaked performance.

As already mentioned, care must be taken not to aggravate pain in what may be already hypersensitised, tense and tender muscles. This situation can be as a result of manual intervention of any type, such as vigorous anal digital (finger) or mechanical device massaging, or as a result of performing overly aggressive voluntary pelvic floor muscle contractions.

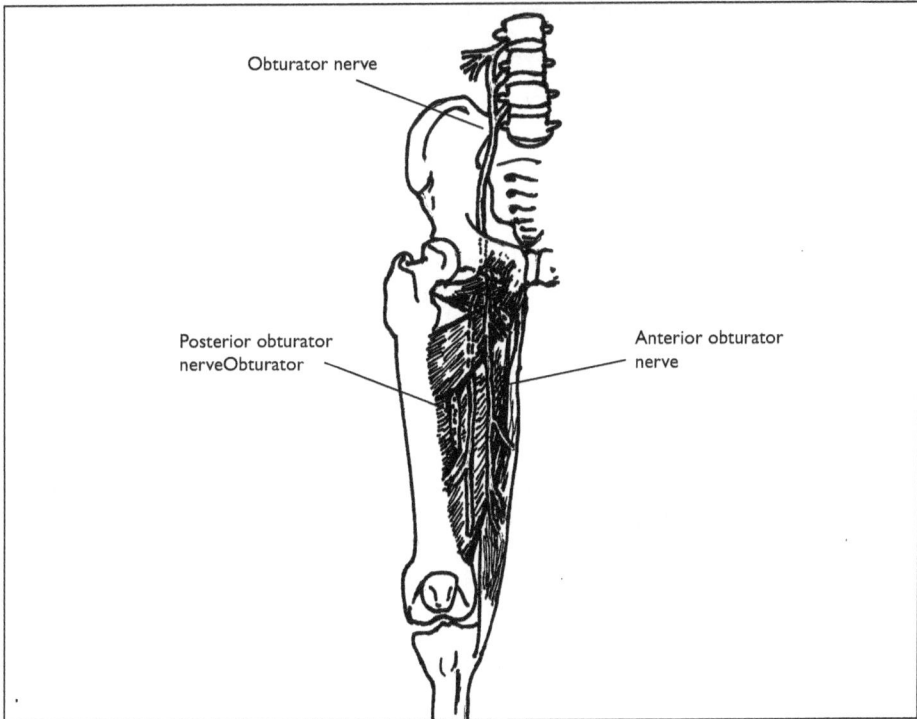

Figure 7b. Obturator Nerve

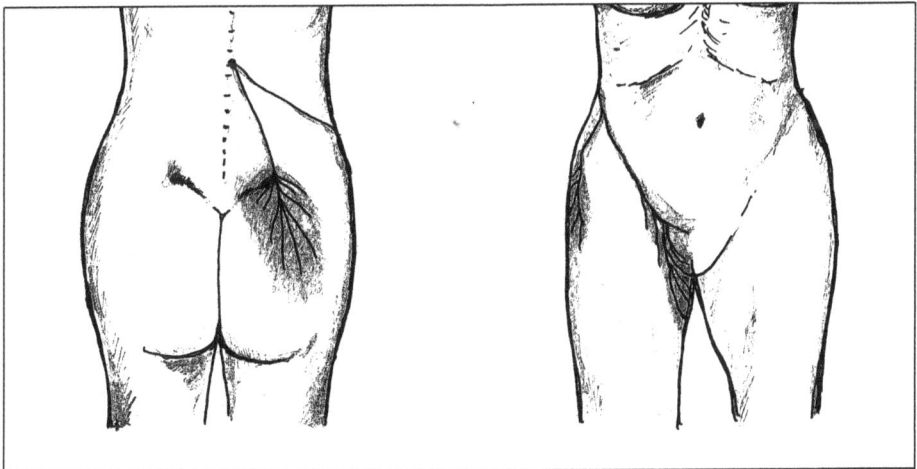

Figure 7c. Maigne's Sydrome

As these muscles are mainly under the control of the pudendal nerve, I find it is *always* more advantageous to search for a primary cause that may compromise the nerve, such as pelvic or sacroiliac dysfunction. If this is the case, address this first.

Overview of Nerve Distribution to Major Anatomical Areas

Penis and clitoris

Shaft and glans (tip of head of penis) and clitoris. Sensation is carried through the penile or clitoral branch (superior or dorsal nerve) of the pudendal nerve. The proximal penis is supplied by the ilioinguinal nerve (L1). The penile urethra is supplied by the inferior pelvic plexus.

Erectile tissue of penis and clitoris

The cavernous nerves (sympathetic system) from the pelvic splanchnic nerves (S2–S4) and the muscular nerve (deep branch) of the perineal branch (inferior nerve) of the pudendal nerve (S2–S4)

Scrotum and labia

- The long scrotal or labial nerve of the perineal branch (inferior nerve) of the pudendal nerve
- Lumbar nerves (iliohypogastric, ilioinguinal, and genitofemoral nerves L1–L2)
- Thoracolumbar junction, T12–L1 (Maigne's Syndrome)
- Posterior femoral cutaneous nerve (S1, S2, S3) via the inferior cluneal nerves

Vulva

External genital organs of female — anterior portion supplied by ilioinguinal nerve (L1) and genital branch of genitofemoral nerve (L1–L2). Posterior portion supplied by pudendal nerve (S2, S3, S4) and inferior cluneal nerves (S1, S2, S3.)

Epididymis and Testes

T10–T11.

Perineum — levator ani and superficial transverse perineal muscles

Muscular nerve (deep branch) of perineal branch (inferior nerve) of pudendal nerve, S2, S3, S4.

Lower part of abdomen

Iliohypogastric, ilioinguinal and genitofemoral nerve L1–L2.

Base of bladder and urethral sphincter

For urge incontinence, suprapubic pain, and voiding problems. Muscular nerve (deep branch) of perineal branch (inferior nerve) of pudendal nerve, S2, S3, S4.

Prostate and upper part of bladder

Inferior hypogastric plexus, T10–L2.

Anus

For faecal urgency and pain at external sphincter and skin around the anus — from the posterior branch of the cutaneous nerve (long scrotal and labial nerve) of the pudendal nerve and the inferior rectal (haemorrhoid) nerve, S2, S3, S4.

Ischial tuberosity

Skin below the ischial tuberosity and to perineum — from the perineal branch of the inferior cluneal nerve from the posterior femoral cutaneous nerve, S1, S2, S3.

Coccyx

Sensory innervation of the skin in the coccygeal region is supplied by the coccygeal plexus, S4, S5 and Co1. The only nerve in this plexus is called the anococcygeal nerve. (Pain here is often misdiagnosed as coccydynia or strained sacrococcygeal ligament).

Upper and Inner parts of the thigh

The lumbar nerves (L1 and L2) — iliohypogastric, ilioinguinal and genitofemoral. Also T12–L1 junction and the sensory branches of the obturator nerve L2–L4.

Erectile Function

Importantly, the pudendal nerve is also vital for erectile function in both sexes. It innervates the corpus cavernosum and corpus spongiosum muscles, which pump blood into the penis to attain an erection, and bulbospongiosus and ischiocavernous muscles, which maintain blood in the penis during erection, while in the female it is used for clitoral erection. It is also involved with the mechanics of defaecation, ejaculation and most of the feelings of orgasm. **Orgasmic sensations** are thought to be shared between the pudendal, pelvic and vagal nerves. (Even though the actual nerve allowing orgasm comes from T11, T12, if the penis is numb [through pudendal nerve damage], sensory messages cannot get through] and orgasm [and ejaculation] cannot occur.)

The nerve is also critical for normal bladder and bowel functions, receiving both visceral and muscular fibres. Depending on the site of damage to the nerve, involvement here can lead to pain in either or both areas plus urinary and/or faecal incontinence and urge incontinence to either or both.

Chapter 2

Musculoskeletal Assessment

As has been stated, there can be many causes of pelvic pain. It is possible
a significant percentage of these can be attributed to compromise of
the pudendal nerve. Revealing an accurate diagnosis may initially
involve a multifaceted approach. This may include assessments and investigations
by health professionals from urology, gynaecology, gastroenterology, neurology,
pain management, pelvic floor physiotherapists and recently from professionals
with a special interest in musculoskeletal health.

Once medical practitioners have cleared the cause as not being related to
something local or systemic, or something that they can treat, the patient should
be referred to a musculoskeletal therapist for further examination.

It is important to be alert to the previous section on musculoskeletal conditions highlighted by Prendergast and Rummer (see page 10), which could
potentially be associated with pudendal neuralgia. However, I strongly recom-
mend, initially, the therapist search for clues implicating lumbar-pelvic
dysfunction, in particular, malalignment of either of the innominates on the
sacrum. What we are searching for is evidence that one or both of the innominates may be significantly rotated on the sacrum, a situation that may cause
compression or traction to be placed on the pudendal nerve.

There is an admitted risk with this direct approach that the therapist may
invoke 'confirmational bias' — that is, you may find what you are searching for.

A certain percentage of the population probably has a degree of pelvic dysfunction and does not demonstrate either lower back pain or pudendal neuralgia symptoms. However, the risk is justified by the research documented in the author's research article referenced in the Introduction.

Theoretically, a strong enough force on the pelvis in *any* direction could change the mechanics in relation to the path of the nerve. Realistically, the most common force that will do this is one that posteriorly rotates the innominate on the sacrum, such as in sitting or during an event that causes extreme flexion of the lower extremity (See Figure 8).

Patient History

As with all assessments *the history* of the patient can reveal important indications. Initially, listen calmly without provocation or leading. This may be the tenth time the patient has repeated his or her story to a health professional, but you may be the first to look for musculoskeletal involvement. It is important to ask some precise questions at the right time.

If the patient presents with, for instance, scrotal pain (or labia pain for women) as 80% of pudendal neuralgia patients do, ask, in order: have they any penile (or clitoral) pain, erectile dysfunction, pain during or after ejaculation (or orgasm), pain on penetration, pain after micturition, urinary urgency or fre-

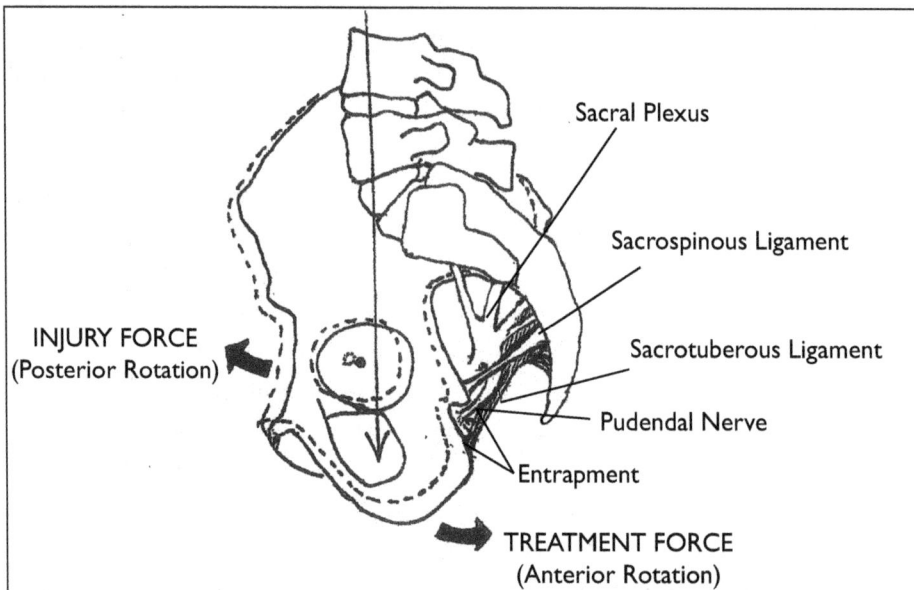

Figure 8. Mechanism of Injury

quency, slowness or inability to void bladder, pain in perineum or pelvic floor region, anal pain either at the sphincter or skin around the anal region, pain after defaecation or faecal urgency, priapism (persistent erection) or genital arousal (without desire). All, or any variation of these, can be symptoms of pudendal neuralgia, which the patient may have not considered to be related to each other. (**Note:** Other nerves can also be involved.) Ask also of a history of lower back pain, with or without referral/sciatic symptoms.

If any of these symptoms are notably worsened by sitting, and particularly if they are accompanied by lower back pain, with or without referral symptoms, these are definite markers to search for a musculoskeletal cause.

So, as such, be alert for clearly relevant histories, ones that involve pelvic rotation, such as:

- An event involving fast, violent action that could rotate either of the innominates on the sacrum such as experiencing a 'jink' in his or her back, an effect similar to that caused by stepping on a stair that's 'not there' or is lower than expected, or jumping off a train or bus. Patients often recall a sensation like a lightning electrical shock.

- Activities involving deceleration, changing direction or swivelling on one foot. Such movements, which could occur during a game of squash, tennis, soccer — (in fact, all high impact sports, including basketball, volleyball etc.). The reality here is that the patient may not immediately have associated this event with his or her pudendal neuralgia symptoms. Further, the patient may not have actually felt any significant back pain at the time, being generally warmed up, focussed and pumping adrenaline. During the incident, there may have been an awareness of something 'going', but only later may actual back pain be experienced, if at all; low-grade, strong, protective muscle spasm of the erector spinae and hip flexor muscles often mask any significant signs of back pain and potential sacroiliac joint involvement. In fact, the first symptom the patient may experience may be one of the symptoms or signs of pudendal neuralgia, such as scrotal pain, which may have occurred instantly (and not that difficult to relate to the particular event), or most often, some days or weeks later (which is more difficult to relate to pelvic involvement or a particular event). It is proposed that this is because the damaged SIJ is maintained in a malaligned position by the stiffening of fibrous tissue at the SIJ. A common presentation here is of tight iliopsoas muscles, tight piriformis muscles and tight, spasmed pelvic floor muscles.

Careful questioning is needed here to match the onset of the symptoms with a possible causative event and/or back pain.

- Bending down quickly to pick up something off the floor, tying up shoe laces, bending over in the garden, cleaning, vacuuming or pushing a shopping trolley.

- The previous cause could be exacerbated by lifting something while bending over, such as tables, chairs, computers, cabinets, gardening pots and shovelling, etc., or grandparents picking up a child (untrained and unfit for the event).

- Sitting can bring on and/or exacerbate symptoms. This can especially affect people who sit for long periods of time, particularly if they do so without an appropriate lumbar support. IT workers and many office workers often sit for ten hours a day without adequate breaks, as do pilots, truck, taxi and courier drivers, and addicted television viewers. A percentage of these people will be overweight and unfit, increasing the potential to rotate and stress the joints.

- Motor vehicle accidents involving severe trauma to the pelvis, causing fractures, dislocations and rotations. Similarly, falls off bicycles (or any fall, for that matter), onto the pelvis, back, hip. A fall onto the knee can also transfer forces to the SIJ resulting in joint damage and subsequent restrictions.

- Cyclists who spend long periods bending over low handle bars, forcing the innominates into a sustained position of extreme posterior rotation. (**Note:** Any pudendal nerve involvement in this instance is different from that caused by sitting on an ill-fitting bicycle seat, which may compress the penile branch of the pudendal nerve against the ischial ramus of the pelvis. The symptom in this case is generally numbness or pain in the penis and is initially treated by cessation of cycling or changing the seat.)

- Sports involving extreme flexion of the spine, such as performing deep squats with heavy weights. This can cause the innominate to excessively posteriorly rotate on the sacrum.

- Sex. Violent, athletic and extreme actions, particularly during orgasm, causing the innominates to excessively rotate on the sacrum.

- Surgery. It is possible to inadvertently place severe rotatory stress on the sacroiliac joint during any surgery where the pelvic girdle has been sustained in an extreme or unsupported position, especially lithotomy position. (**Note:** Surgery can also compromise the pudendal nerve from incisions, compression from retractors, suture ligature and scarring. These causes **won't** be assisted by pelvic dysfunction treatment.)

- This previous situation, of course, can also occur during exhaustive sleep, or whilst under the influence of drugs or alcohol. In these cases, an individual can suffer any type and degree of neuropathy, particularly palsy to nerves of the brachial or sciatic plexuses. (During healthy sleep, nature intends an individual to roll or change position 40 to 50 times a night in order to take stress off muscles, tendons, ligaments, blood vessels, nerves, etc.). As with the effects of anaesthetics during surgery, in these situations, it is possible to compromise the pudendal nerve as the dead weight of the body can place exceptional pressure on the sacroiliac joints.

- The pudendal nerve symptoms are often associated with and accompanied by lower back pain, buttocks, and thigh or leg pain. This lower back pain and limb pain is generally a somatic referred pain. Somatic pain is generated from a somatic structure (joint, muscle tendon, disc). The pain is often deep and hard to localise and can move from area to area. This is unlike radicular pain, which is due to irritation of a spinal nerve root or dorsal root ganglion. The most common cause of radicular pain is an acute disc prolapse, which will generally start in the buttock and can be a normal non-dermatonal line from start to finish.

Sometimes, on questioning, the patient can recall that both the pudendal neuralgia symptoms and back symptoms started at about the same time, but it is rare for them to have previously connected their possible relationships. Most times, the stress on the innominates and sacroiliac joints have been slow and subtle (years of sitting incorrectly perhaps), that significant lower back pain does not always occur.

In fact, for many situations, no matter what the cause, low-grade muscular spasm may protect the back against pain. This muscle spasm, hypertonus, triggers articular-muscular reflexes, which maintain the erector muscles in a sustained poor postural position. Further, sometimes the original traumatising event may have occurred so long ago (many years) that the back (SIJ) injury will have healed and the resultant fibrous tissue will have stiffened, also helping to maintain the joint in a restricted position. This can occur to the extent where the patient does not necessarily, at this stage, complain of back pain. He or she may not even complain of stiffness, but that is what your further examination and questioning will search for — SIJ back pain and/or stiffness.

Physical Assessment

Researchers have consistently reported that the clinical diagnosis of symptomatic SIJ remains problematic. Although they concede that sacroiliac joint pain is common in patients with lower back pain, they believe it can only be definitively diagnosed using diagnostic local anaesthetic blocks. However, there is agreement that combined provocative clinical tests may be useful.

One of the problems appears to be that most provocative clinical tests evaluate either function or pain, which of course, may not equate to each other, and certainly may not adequately equate to SIJ damage consistent to trigger a varied plethora of pudendal neuralgia symptoms.

My experience is that most patients who present with a diagnosis of pudendal neuralgia, (which has not been attributed to an obvious urological, gynaecological, gastroenterological or neurological cause), may, on examination, be found to have either SIJ pain and/or dysfunction, or both. However, vexingly, some patients, particularly patients with chronic pudendal neuralgia symptoms, may be found to have no SIJ pain, and only minimal dysfunction, often so minimal that they have not been aware of it.

Sometimes, testing may reveal tight iliopsoas muscles, piriformis tension and tight, painful pelvic floor muscles. Digital massage and relaxation techniques can often relieve some of these symptoms, but I have observed rarely relieves the pudendal neuralgia symptoms. (In fact, because the pelvic floor muscles are supplied by the pudendal nerve, trigger point massage often exacerbates symptoms.) Therefore, I consider that in some cases, ones where provocative clinical tests do not reveal significant pain and/or dysfunction, another criterion must be introduced.

What I propose now arises from a purely clinical observation. I submit that what we really have to look for here is SIJ **stiffness** — often so little stiffness that it may not show up effectively with any pain, functional or provocative tests.

As previously proposed, I consider for the SIJ to be involved in the cause of pudendal neuralgia, where one (or both) of the innominates has to be appreciably restricted in its movement on the sacrum. In this regard, the patient's **history** may already have alerted us and revealed perhaps a pertinent specific event, or the use of a habitual poor seating posture, which may be associated with this possibility.

Therefore, with all this in mind, the real key, I believe, to implicate SIJ involvement is to search for joint stiffness. This is done by using palpation to thoroughly explore the joint. It is not dissimilar to classic 'spring tests' used for motion grading to test actual mobility in the joint.

If the injury is significant, such as related to a specific, notable event, and recent (within six weeks), palpation over the SIJ will generally be reactive, painful and stiff. However, if the examination is carried out many months, or even years, after the causative event, the body (and brain) may have adapted to this new situation and clinically, there may be no notable dysfunction or pain. The only finding may be localised joint stiffness, which may only be revealed on sensitive and creative palpation. Generally, this will be a posterior to anterior glide force of about 10 pounds (about 4.7 kilograms) to take up the slack, then an additional 10 pounds to 'spring' or get to the 'end feel'.[1]

I have found it useful to refer to Maitland's[2] classic mobilisation grading.

I note degrees of pain and stiffness as:

Grade I — small amplitude

Grade II — larger amplitude

For stiffness only — no irritability

Grade III — large amplitude

Grade IV — small end of range-of-movement amplitude

This, of course, is useful for recording the status of the joint at the initial assessment, and also for acknowledging the effectiveness of ongoing treatment.

A small warning here: Some patients with chronic pelvic pain symptoms who have been on various medications for pain relief (and for other comorbidities such as high cholesterol, etc.) can present with a swollen, often bloated abdomen. Initially, be aware that aggressive palpation over the SIJ may inflame symptoms.

To appreciate the rationale for, and the validity of this test, a deeper understanding of the process of the pathology of healing and regeneration, as discussed briefly in Chapter 1, is necessary. Simply, in the early inflammatory and fibroblastic phases of healing, usually the first few weeks, fibroblasts replace the damaged ligaments with fibrous tissue and aggregate into collagen fibres, an activity that may eventually take from six to ten weeks.

As the healing process moves into the final stage, the maturation phase, remodelling of the wound develops the collagen fibres into a stronger weave, a process that may require six to twelve months. This fibrous (scar) tissue, however, is less extensible; the joint becomes stiff, potentially malaligning the innominate on the sacrum. (Of importance, experience and documentation has shown that it is possible to minimise the negative effects of this process. Early intervention such as appropriate exercise and mobilisation can influence and control fibrosis and limit dysfunction by remodelling and 'unwinding' the scar tissue fibres.)

When testing for stiffness, it is important to remember that motion of the **pelvic girdle is** a triplanar movement. That is, movement can occur in all three body planes — flexion/extension, side flexion and axial rotations — producing potential for six degrees of freedom. However, as noted earlier, the SIJ is only capable of limited rotational and translational movement in one plane. Therefore, it is not difficult to imagine how, when **great** stress is applied from any of the above-mentioned planes, theoretically, any part or combination of parts of any of the ligaments that stabilise the SIJ could be injured.

Further, the SIJ is L-shaped, much like a boomerang with one arm shorter than the other. Therefore, it is important to thoroughly search and palpate in any and every direction you can creatively manage. (Keep in mind, as mentioned earlier, the joint can exhibit two, or even three, planes of movement.)

When stiffness is found, this situation is often referred to as the joint being 'out', 'malaligned', 'fixated', or 'excessively compressed'.

The other area that is useful to test is the coccyx. While a fall on the coccyx can potentially rotate the sacrum on the innominate, it can also strain or dislocate the coccyx on the sacrum, damaging the connecting ligaments. As fibres from both the sacrotuberous and sacrospinous ligaments attach to the coccyx, and the pudendal nerve moves between the sacrotuberous and sacrospinous ligaments, it is possible to create significant compression on the pudendal nerve.

If the coccyx area itself is painful, it is important to test the sacrococcygeal symphysis ligaments by palpation for pain and/or stiffness. However, in my experience, most pain in the coccyx area is referred from the anococcygeal nerve (S4, S5, Co1), which can be compromised by sacroiliac joint dysfunction, so also test for sacroiliac joint stiffness, pain or dysfunction.

Chapter 3

Treatment

The musculoskeletal treatment to manage symptoms of pudendal neuropathy, particularly in relation to the SIJ, is approached in four phases:

1. The primary aim of treatment is to release the restrictions maintaining the innominate on the sacrum in an incorrect position. This is achieved initially by manual mobilising and manipulative techniques, then maintained by exercises.

2. It is imperative to teach the patient how to maintain the correct and optimal lumbar posture, particularly whilst sitting.

3. There may be a need to understand and manage chronic pain cycles and neural hypersensitivity.

4. A prevention program should be instituted by maintaining an appropriate exercise program and being constantly aware of the importance of correct posture.

Releasing the Restrictions Maintaining the Innominate in an Incorrect Position on the Sacrum

There are many possible presentations of SIJ dysfunction (involving abnormal rotation of the innominate on the sacrum), that may cause pudendal neuropathy, pudendal neuralgia or pudendal nerve entrapment and its associated symptoms. The immediate aim of treatment in all cases is to realign the innominate on the sacrum.

It must be noted here that a common presentation of SIJ dysfunction is tight iliopsoas and hip flexors and weak gluteals and hamstrings. The immediate tendency for treatment is to stretch the iliopsoas and hip flexor muscles. However, as this joint is the strongest joint in the body and has evolved to keep us erect, as a rule, no amount of active stretching exercises will mobilise or have a significant impact on changing the alignment of the joint.

The only effective way to mobilise the SIJ is by manual techniques.

The most common presentation is one where the innominate is rotated posteriorly on the sacrum (See Figure 8 back on page 38.). The aim of treatment, in this case, is to 'realign' the innominate by rotating it anteriorly. This is achieved in three stages; (i), heating the SIJ tissues, (ii) mobilising the sacroiliac joint manually and (iii) exercising.

Heat

Heat is applied to the SIJ and to the tissues in the surrounding areas. The main effects of heat, in this instance, are:

- To relieve pain in the joint and the surrounding tissues. It is found that a mild degree of heating is effective in relieving pain, presumably as a result of a sedative effect on the sensory nerves.

- To relieve protective muscle spasm. By virtue of relieving pain, associated muscle spasm and tension are also relieved.

- To increase extensibility of the collagen fibres of the scar tissue of the SIJ that is maintaining the innominate in the incorrect position. When considering the reaction of heat on soft tissue, it has been shown that temperature has a significant influence on the mechanical behaviour of connective tissue under tensile stress. As tissue temperature rises, stiffness decreases and extensibility increases. Both applied heat and exercise can produce a temperature rise.

- To enhance easier mobilising/stretching routines and to facilitate muscle contractility.

In the therapists' rooms, shortwave and microwave diathermy penetrate deeply and produce as much as five to six degrees increase in temperature to a depth of 5 cm. At home, heat packs, infrared lamp, hot-water bag, warm showers and baths are all effective.

Mobilisation — Manual mobilising and manipulative techniques

Basically, the term mobilisation refers to a stretching process designed to increase the range of movement of a stiff joint. It is a collective term incorporating two techniques, mobilisation and manipulation. Mobilisation can be applied as passive small or large oscillatory movements, two or three a second, anywhere in a range of movement, and it can also be applied as a sustained stretch at the limit of the range. Manipulation describes a sudden movement or thrust, of small amplitude and high speed, at the end of the range.

Mobilisation can be achieved by the therapist manually by applying 'passive movement' techniques to the joint (See Figure 9), or by the patient actively performing specific exercises.

For the SIJ the aim of mobilisation is to restore structures within the joint to their normal position so as to recover a full-range painless movement.

Initially, once the therapist has identified specific stiff structures within the SIJ, small amplitude passive movement techniques are used to mobilise the SIJ. As the joint does not move around a single, clearly defined axis, this will take some creativity. The therapist must search for stiff sections in all ligamentous, fibrotic and fascial structures and tissues that make up the SIJ. This will include any spin, roll or slide features that are normal for the joint. This will also mean searching for, and mobilising, any adaptive stiffening of any other related joint structures.

As the joint shows signs that this technique is gradually increasing mobility, the therapist may then introduce a slow, stronger, stretching technique holding in a sustained position for about 10–15 seconds, building up to at least a minute, even two minutes. Do not stint on time or pressure here. We are trying to change the quality of scar tissue restrictions by utilising principles of viscoelastic creep[1]. Creep is an important concept when treating isolated SIJ mobility. It is known that treatment forces held steady against a motion barrier (adhesions, spasm) for several minutes will induce tissue relaxation resulting in an increase in joint mobility and soft-tissue extensibility. The tissue is taken beyond the elastic limit inducing plastic (more lasting) deformation. Clinically, the scarring is fundamentally altered. A special technique for this presentation is to stretch the SIJ by rotating the innominate anteriorly (See Figure 9).

With the patient lying prone close to the edge of the table, the therapist supports the anterior aspect of the distal thigh with one hand and lifts the hip into extension, while the posterior superior iliac spine of the innominate is palpated with the heel of the other hand. The limit of anterior rotation of the innominate is reached by passively extending the hip with one hand and applying an anterior rotation force to the innominate with the other hand. The pressure is held for 15 seconds, building up to a minute or more on full stretch.

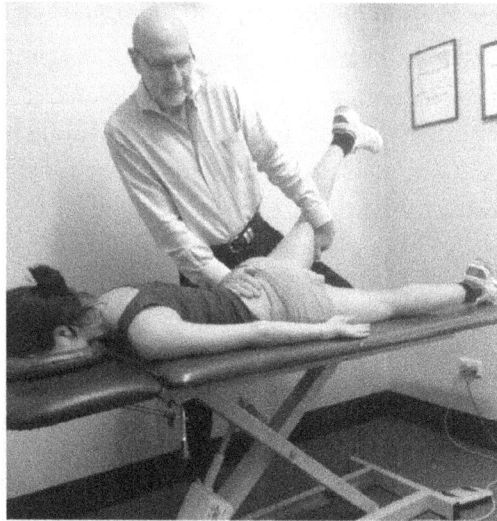

Figure 9. Manual Mobilising Stretch

This effect can be enhanced by applying a manipulative technique to the SIJ. (see Figure 10). With the patient in right-side lying, lower leg extended and upper hip and knee flexed, the thoracolumbar spine is fully rotated to the left. Find the stiffest level of resistance. The therapist stabilises the sacrum with one hand while the other hand applies a high-velocity, low-amplitude thrust through the left innominate.

An instructional video for therapists on how to perfrom this manipulation is available from the author's website — www.peterdornanphysio.com.au.

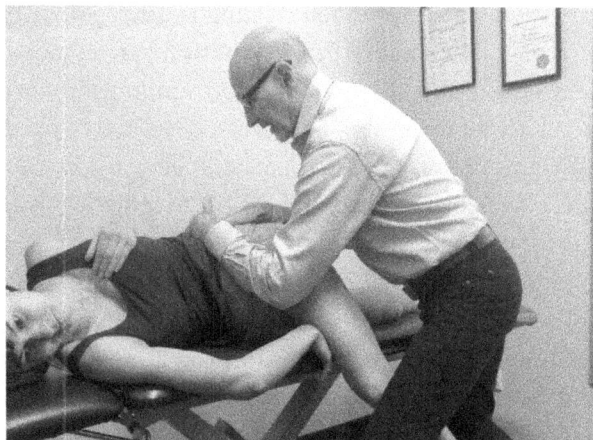

Figure 10. Manipulation of the SIJ — Posterior Distraction of the Left SIJ

Although researchers are not sure of the exact mechanism underlying the effects of this technique, it is considered to be effective to restore joint mobility, for whatever reason.[2]

Exercises

Exercises are important. Because the ligaments of the SIJ and the lumbar spine mesh with the thoracolumbar fascia, and are the primary attachments for the stabilisers of the spine, exercises are designed not just to maintain the joint range of movement or to regain the flexibility, strength and endurance components of the muscles that control the joint, but to restimulate joint and muscle mechanoreceptors. The following exercises should be performed at least once a day. As scarring contracts/stiffens with inactivity, the injured areas will generally be at their stiffest first thing in the morning. This is the recommended time to run through the exercises.

Hip Rolls (See Figure 11)

Patient lying supine, legs hip-width apart, lift the buttocks to a long diagonal line between the shoulders, hips and knees. Roll or glide the pelvis to one side, back to the middle, then the other. Return to the middle and lower buttocks to the floor. 10 repetitions.

Lower Back Stretch (see Figure 12)

Patient lying supine, use two hands to draw one thigh and knee to the chin, keeping the other leg flat and extended. Hold this thigh on strong overpressure for 5 seconds and release. Repeat 5 repetitions each leg.

Full-Spine Strengthening (see Figure 13)

Patient kneeling on all fours, hands underneath shoulders, knees under hips, flex and stretch one knee towards the chin, then extend head and leg. Repeat 10 times for each leg, building up to 3 sets of 10 repetitions. As the patient adapts to this routine, an ankle weight should be added to the ankle to increase resistance.

SIJ Stretch (see Figure 14a & 14b)

Patient kneeling on a chair with elbows placed on strong table. One leg (knee) is positioned over the edge of the chair and hooked over the other leg for support. (a) The aforementioned leg is stretched fully below the edge of the chair and held in position here for 5 seconds, then (b) lifted fully higher than the edge of the chair and held here for five seconds. This is repeated on each side 10 times.

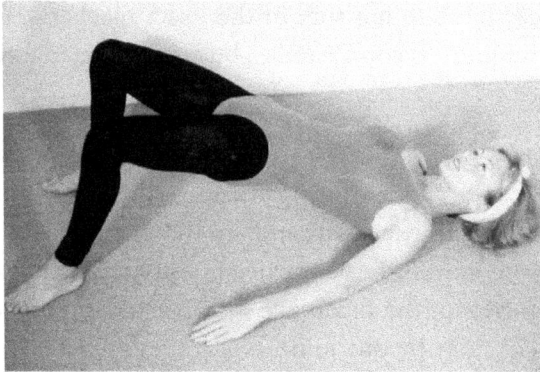

Figure 11. Hip Rolls

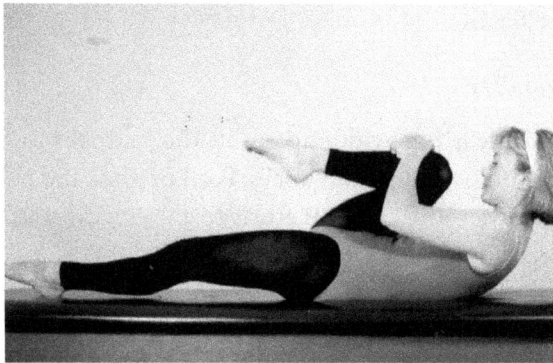

Figure 12. Low Back Stretch

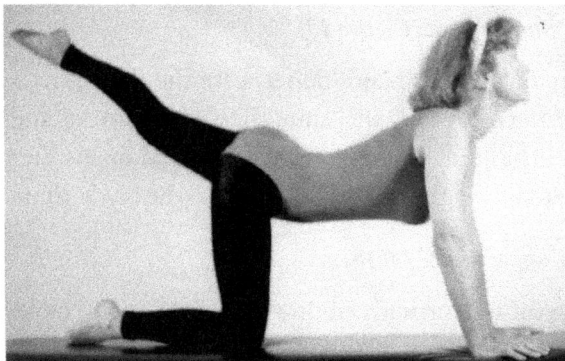

Figure 13. Full Spine Strengthening

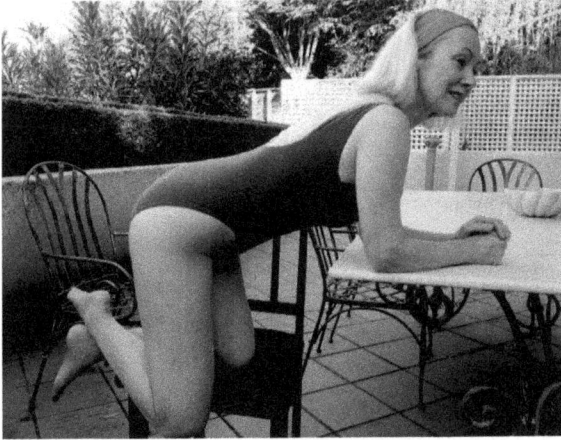

Figure 14a. SIJ Stretch

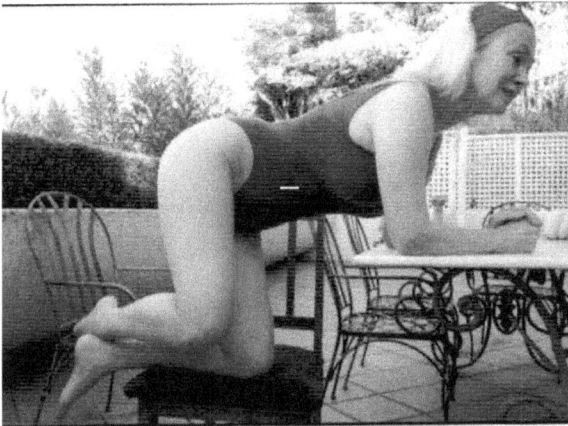

Figure 14b. SIJ Stretch

Abdominal (Core) Exercises (see Figures 15 a & 15b)

Patient in supine, knees flexed, feet flat on floor, hands behind head and neck supported. Draw the navel to the floor to flatten abdominals, and then raise head and shoulders (as in 'crunches'). Repeat 6 times. Then, as the patient sits up, rotate the trunk towards one knee, repeat 6 times. Repeat to the other knee 6 times.

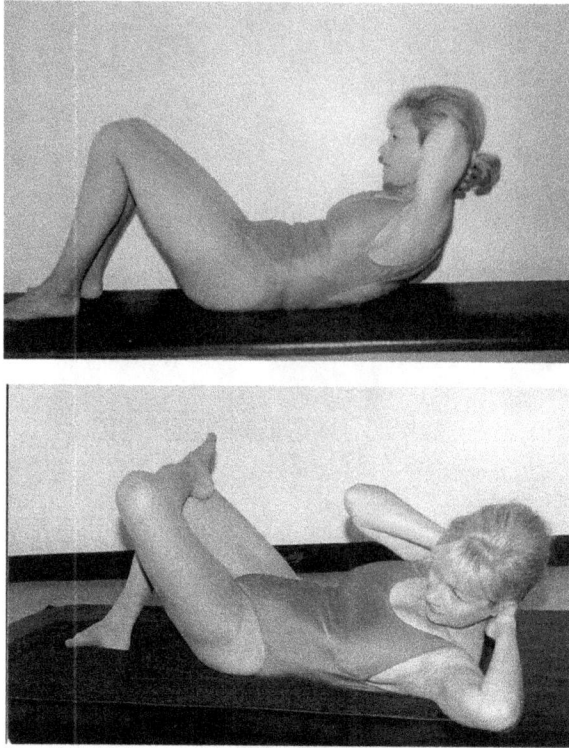

Figure 15. a & b. Abdominal (core) Exercises

Maintaining the Correct Lumbar Posture

Incorrect posture, particularly in sitting, is probably the major underlying cause of the endemic incidence of spinal pain in Western society. It can certainly be the cause of certain presentations of pudendal neuropathy. By the time we reach our late thirties, the physical consequences of a lifetime of sedentary occupations, particularly IT related, hobbies, and television habits become obvious.

There's a curve to our posture that wasn't there before. The head begins to slump forward, changing the entire balance of the body. The head weighs 5 kg. This is the amount of stress placed on the neck when the head is perched squarely on a person with good posture while standing erect (Figure 16). When the head slumps forward 2 cms, the stress on the neck doubles — when it slumps forward 4 cms, it quadruples — effectively increasing the stress on the neck to 20 kg.

Our shoulders become more rounded. Our chest, or breasts (which can weigh 2–3 kg each) sag, our belly protrudes, and to compensate for the weight of the head being pushed forward, the body deepens the curve in the lumbar spine, increasing stress on it (see Figure 16).

Poor sitting posture reverses the normal curves of the spine in the regions of the neck and lower back. This situation produces a prolonged stretch to the ligaments of the spine. It is like stretching an elastic band to its extreme until it frays, then breaks. This prolonged stretch produces micro-stress trauma to all the soft-tissue spinal structures, and they respond by scarring and shortening (see Figure 17). It is this situation that can stress and damage the sacroiliac joints as the pelvis rotates, forcing the innominates to posteriorly rotate on the sacrum.

Poor posture is becoming increasingly evident in our children and adolescents, particularly in the slouching position they adopt in standing and sitting. Postural defects worsen with age as the effects of sedentary life (lack of exercise, poor diet, overweight, obesity and stress), take their toll.

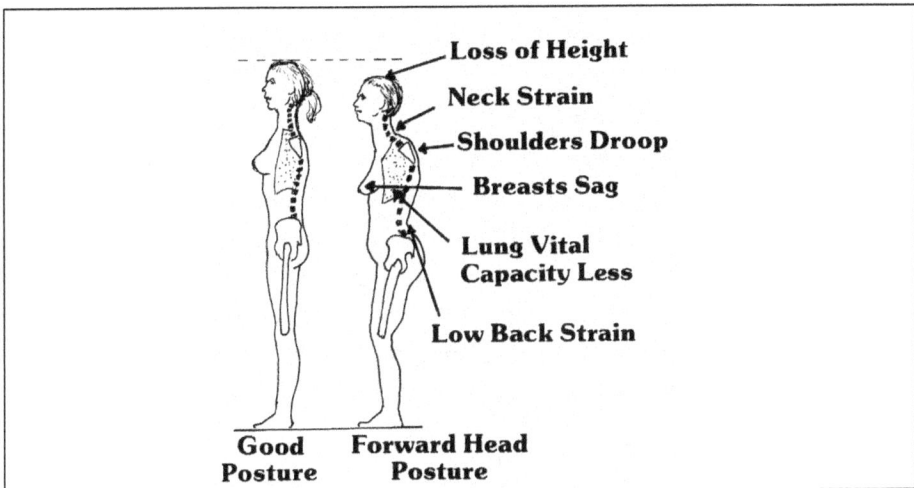

Figure 16. The Importance of Good Posture

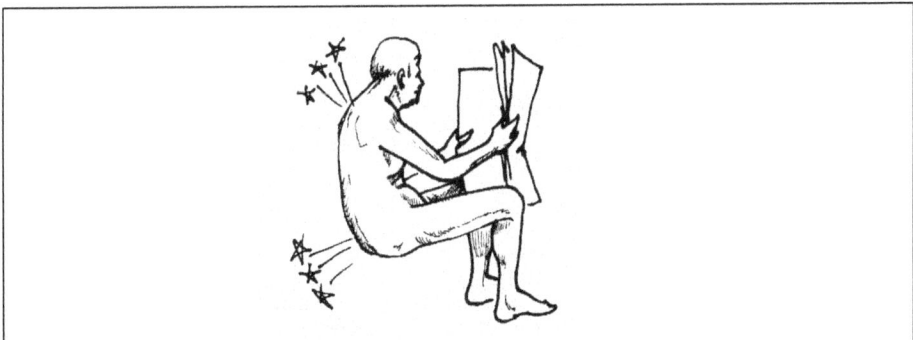

Figure 17. Poor Seating Posture

Note the change from correct posture to poor posture (as in Young Norm) to 40-year-old Norm (see Figure 18). This exaggerated diagram is becoming the caricature of 21st Century Person, the 'Norm' of everyday life.

The postural strategies to manage and prevent symptoms of pudendal neuropathy and pudendal neuralgia are the same as those for managing back pain. It is critical that you become aware of your posture. If you examine your spinal column from the side, you will notice it has evolved to form an efficient spring shape. If this shape is altered extremely, the spine may be injured. **Try to maintain this natural curve in its optimal position during all changes of posture.**

Regaining Correct Posture

After some years of poor postural practices, the brain actually becomes programmed to believe it is normal for the head to be jutting forward, the shoulders to be rounded and the lower back and pelvis to be excessively rotated. The first step in regaining correct posture is to retrain the brain to be aware of where it should be.

All you need to do is STAND TALL. Lift your head and push it to the ceiling (see Figure 18). It's something you can do any time. Have deliberate posture checks regularly — at least twice daily. Think about standing tall. Imagine, if you like, you are balancing a book or weight on the top of your head. Try and keep it high. One of the most effective times to do this is on arising in the morning when joints, muscles and tendons will generally be at their stiffest. As well, write 'P" (for posture) on your desk or watch, or schedule for a regular reminder to be flagged on your computer.

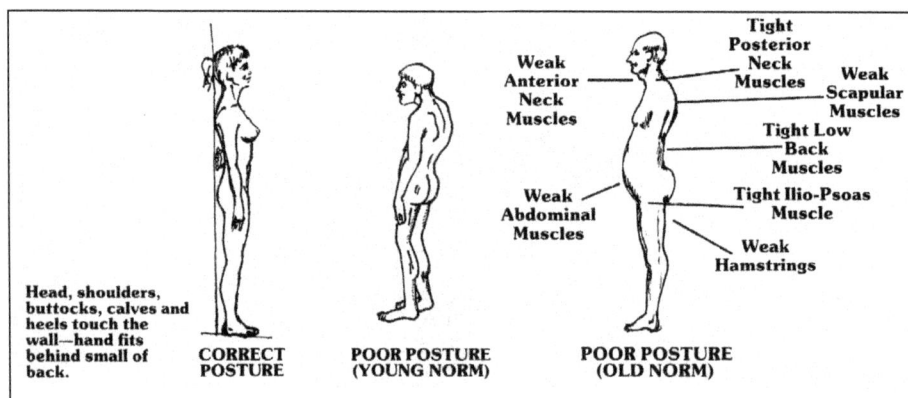

Figure 18. Correct Posture to Poor Posture

Sitting

When sitting, make sure all parts of your lower back and neck are supported. You may have to place a cushion behind your lower back to keep the curve in its natural and optimal shape (see Figure 19). Be sure not to rotate the pelvis excessively in either direction. If the chair is low, and your knees are higher than your buttocks, you may also need to place a cushion under your buttocks. You don't have to use a straight back chair — just a comfortable, supportive one. Do this when driving, watching TV, sitting at work or at home at the dinner table. Further, you are advised to regularly change your posture every 30 minutes, even if you have no pain — stand up and walk around regularly. Keep reminding the brain of correct postural patterns.

Prolonged neck bending can lead to pain and headaches from excess strain and eventually, may lead to early degeneration of the spine. Do not have your head leaning forward for long periods, especially when at the computer, reading or knitting (see Figure 20). Desk and workbench heights must also be arranged to prevent excessive forward tilt of the neck. In general, if your head bends further than 30 degrees forward, you have a greater risk of developing neck pain. Remember the advice at the beginning of this section; it is worth repeating: Your head weighs about 5 kg (12 lb). If your head leans forward 2 cms, the stress on your neck virtually doubles in weight (now 10 kg). If you lean over 4 cms, it quadruples (now 20 kg or 48 lbs). This pressure can eventually be thrust onto your lower back, potentially causing or exacerbating the pudendal nerve symptoms.

When sitting at your computer workstation, your hips should be as far back in your chair as possible (see Figure 21). Adjust the backrest so it fits snugly in

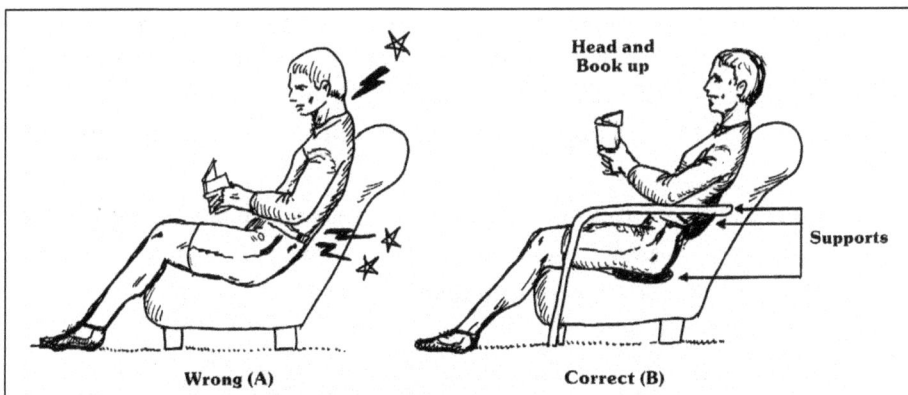

Figure 19. Correct Sitting Posture
[Computer Workstations: Design and adjustment. University of Queensland OHS. 2009]

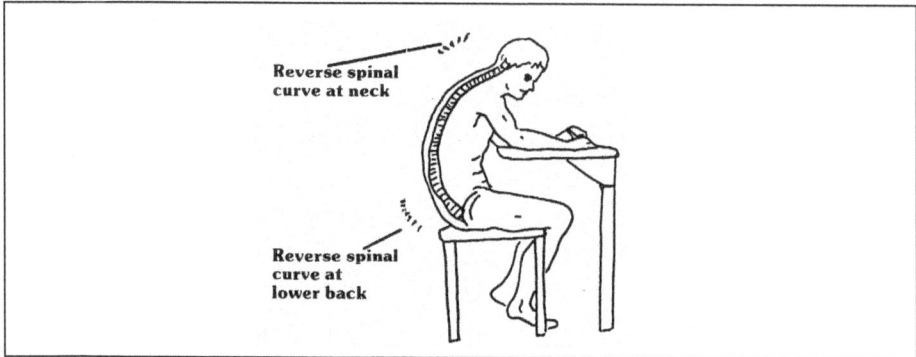

Figure 20. Wrong Desk Posture

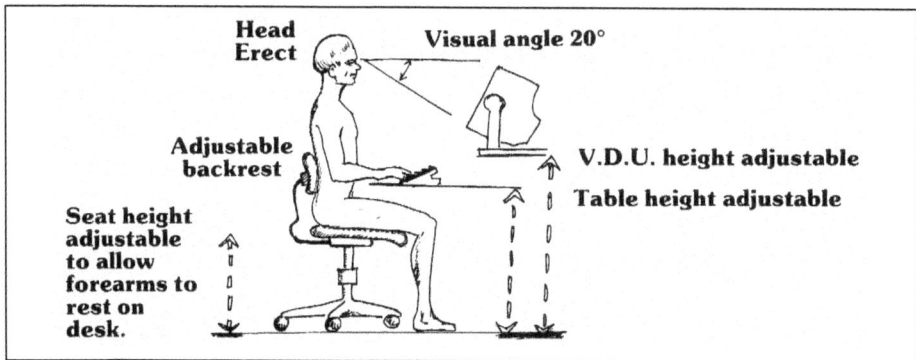

Figure 21. Correct Computer Workstation Posture

the small of your back or use a lumbar roll. Your keyboard should be relatively close to your body and directly in front of you so your forearms rest on the desk. Your seated elbow height should be approximately the same height as the desk. Your neck should be in a neutral position, so place the keyboard and screen directly in front. The optimum position for the computer screen is 15 to 50 degrees below the horizontal line of sight — not at eye level. Your thighs should be parallel to the floor and your knees and ankles should be about 90 degrees.

Your feet should be well supported on the ground. Finally, laptops are difficult to use and maintain correct posture — for sustained periods of comfortable use, limit laptops use, or connect to external screen.

Driving

When driving, there are four main points to follow to prevent neck and back pain.

1. The hip and knees should be parallel to the ground. Often, modern low cars are designed with the front of the seat higher than the back. You may therefore need to add a cushion under your rear to achieve a good driving posture (See Figure 22).

2. Arrange the car seat close to the steering wheel, with the back rest adjusted as near as possible to the upright position.

3. If the seat is fitted with an adjustable lumbar support, this should be positioned to comfortably support the inward curve of the lower back. If there is not adequate lumbar support, use a small pillow, towel or commercial lumbar support. This is critical for managing PN.

4. The steering wheel should be gripped as low down as possible (the recommended safety position is a quarter-to-three; ten-to-two is okay). If the hands are held too high on the wheel, the weight of the arms will quickly overload the neck.

When driving long distances, get out of the car regularly — at least every two hours — and walk around for a minimum of 5 minutes. Stretch the neck and back muscles deliberately. Generally, loosen up body structures and increase circulation.

Sitting on the Toilet

When 'pushing' on the toilet, keep your head up, lean forward a little, take care not to slump and try and maintain the normal lumbar curve (see Figure 23). Place your hands on your knees. Your knees should be slightly higher than your hips. A low footstool can be useful. Relax the lower abdomen first, then further bulge out your abdomen. If you draw the abdomen inward to increase the intra-

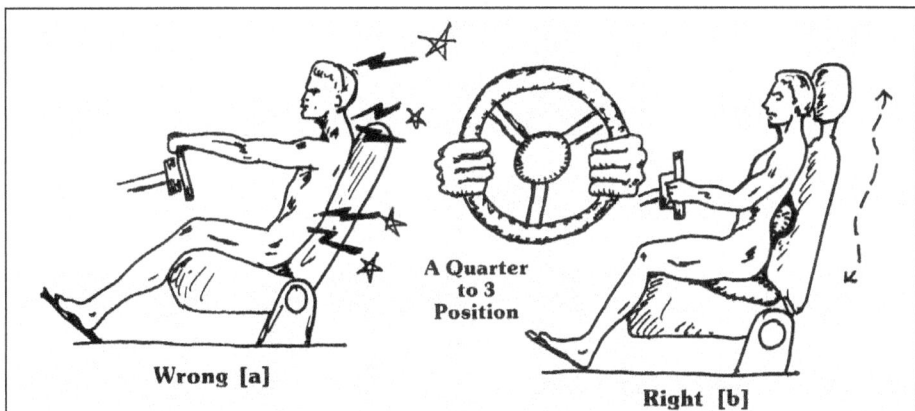

Figure 22. Driving Posture

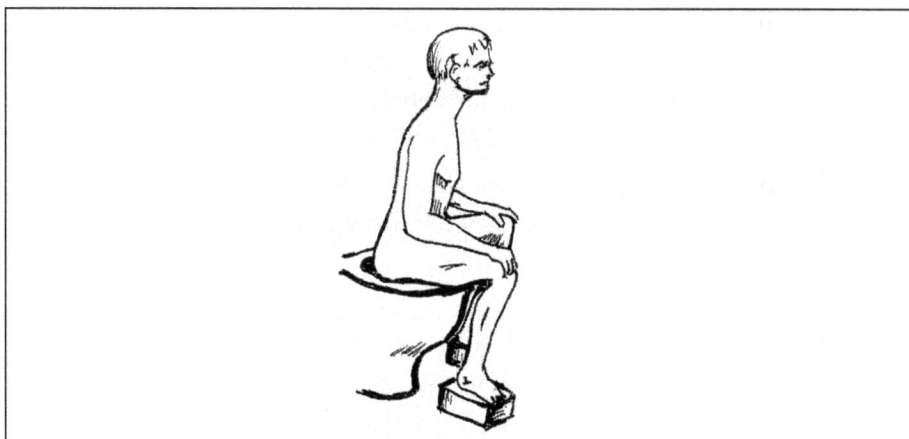

Figure 23. Toilet Posture

abdominal pressure to defaecate, the pelvic floor muscles automatically draw upwards. As the pudendal nerve supplies the pelvic floor muscles, this can trigger pain. So, it is important to relax both the pelvic floor muscles and the abdominal muscles. Sometimes it is helpful to massage the abdomen, applying strong pressure following the intestines to the bowel.

Standing

Prolonged standing in one position places great pressure on the lumbar spine. Shifting the weight from one foot to the other relieves this strain. At the hotel bar, keep a foot on the rail or a rung of the bar stool. Similarly, use a footrest whilst ironing (see Figure 24).

Sneezing, Coughing

Sneeze or cough upwards, (taking care not to cough on anyone), rather than bending forward and risking placing increased intra-abdominal and intra-pelvic pressure on the SIJs. Arch your spine backwards and, placing your hands in the small of your back, push in to equalise the pressure as you cough and sneeze (see Figure 25).

Heavy Loads

Heavy loads should be balanced on both shoulders. If the package cannot be divided, it should be switched from side to side to relieve the lopsided pressure. (e.g., attaché cases or babies, shopping bags, etc.). Schoolchildren should wear schoolbags or backpacks if possible.

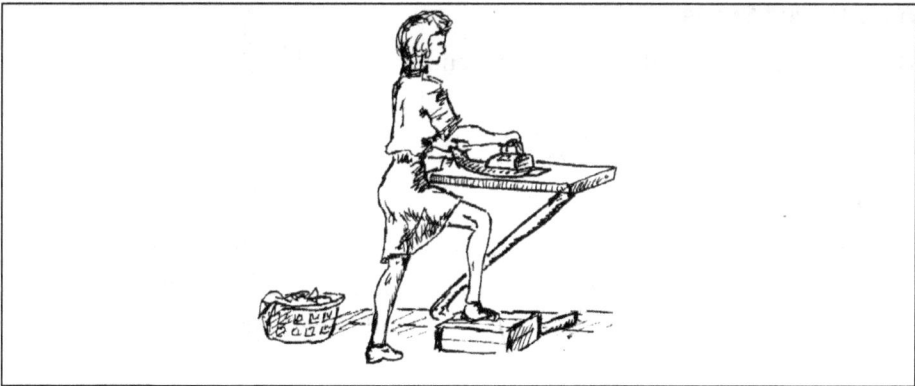

Figure 24. Standing

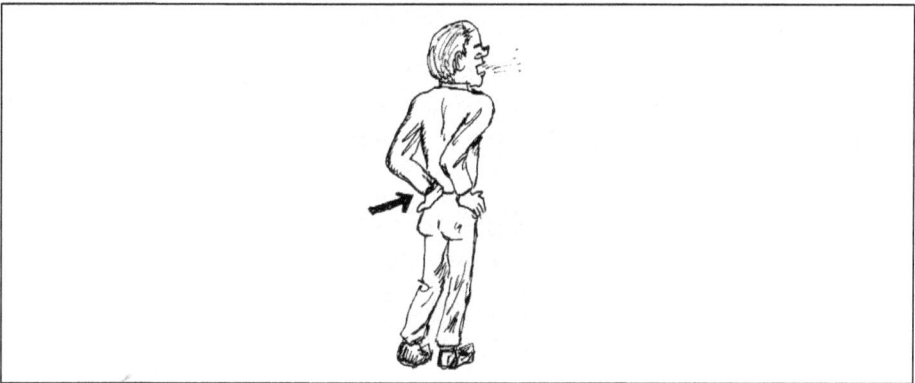

Figure 25. Sneezing, Coughing

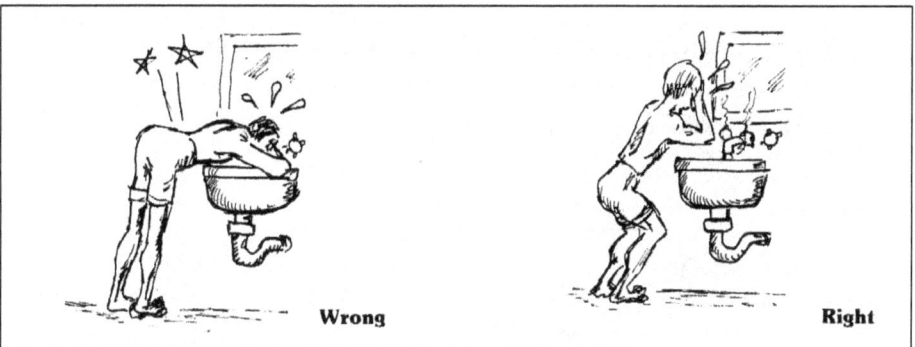

Figure 26. Morning Stiffness

Morning Stiffness

Be careful bending over the sink for a wash first thing in the morning. The back may be stiff from sleeping — scar tissue has a tendency to contract, deform and stiffen with immobility. Maintain the lower back hollow and bend the knees. (See Figure 26).

High-Heeled Shoes

Be wary of high-heeled shoes, as they tend to throw the spine forward by tilting the pelvis. The price of fashion does not always outweigh the price of stress to the SIJ.

Gardening

When gardening and digging, take the strain with your legs and not your back. Use a longer handled spade or shovel to prevent bending the back. Do not bend over while weeding. Use your whole body and kneel close to the weeds, loosening the soil first.

Lifting

When lifting, bend the knees and take the weight through the thigh muscles — they are stronger than the back. The back is not a crane. Get as close as possible to the object you are lifting, brace your abdominal muscles strongly, keep the back 'straight', (see Figure 27) and lift steadily.

Managing Flare-ups: Neural Hypersensitivity

When managing chronic pelvic pain syndrome (CPPS), it is important to understand that chronic or persistent pain can develop into a disease by itself. In fact, CPPS is complex, involving multiple systems. It is about a dynamic network that includes the central nervous system (CNS), peripheral nervous system (PNS) and the end organ. Therefore, a multidisciplinary approach may be required. A diagnosis is often reached by exclusion. We know there are many factors that can potentially interfere with normal pain modulation.

Animals and human beings have developed pain as a warning — an alert concerning a stressful or threatening situation. It is a basic survival mechanism

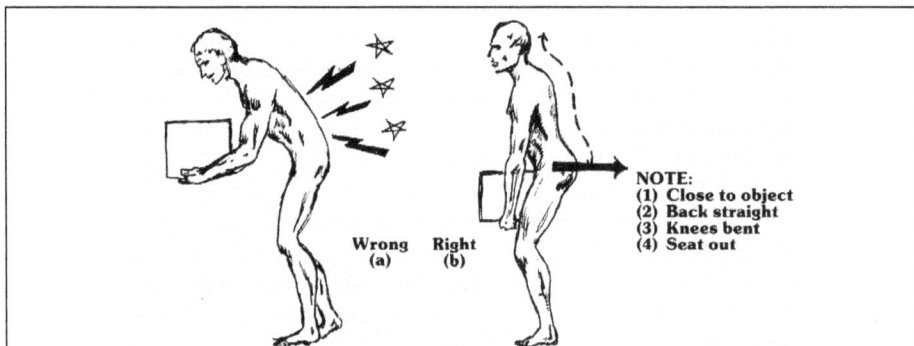

Figure 27. Correct Lifting Procedure

in response to a perception of threat. The process is known as nociception, and it has probably saved you countless of times. When you touch a hot iron, nociceptive receptors funnel messages to your brain, which responds by automatically moving away from the danger — fast. If you sprain an ankle, the pain message to the brain will be perceived as a threat and the responding behaviour to not walk on it and thus aggravate the injury will help it heal.

In the same time, pain (and fear of pain) also triggers the fight or flight reflex. By secreting certain hormones within a few seconds, the body will mobilise all systems to either punch a perpetrator (or move the iron), or run fast from the stressful situation. (In fact, in the case with the iron, nature has developed a short circuit. Instead of having to wait for the message to travel to the spine and then be transferred on to the brain [where the brain can interpret the message, then either consciously consider the threat or spontaneously react], an automatic reflex — a short circuit working locally in the spine — directs us to act quickly. Then the hormones kick in to allow us to challenge, or not, what was threatening us.)

This is pain working naturally and appropriately. Once the threatening situation has been removed, the adrenaline settles down and the painful proactive reflex cycle diminishes.

However, in the case of CPPS, there is generally an ongoing input from a persistent focus; the obstruction or stimulant causing the pain doesn't go away. If the offending structure such as (in our alleged case) an extremely rotated pelvis, (which presumably then exerts pressure on the pudendal nerve), isn't diagnosed and therefore not adequately treated, a chronic pain cycle may develop.

This is when pain does not react appropriately. It becomes a mind/body disorder, a behavioural state with multidisciplinary connections. As stated earlier, chronic pain is complex. It does not necessarily correlate with the degree of injury or disease; it is completely real and is indistinguishable from the original pain when the nerve was originally assaulted. Psychosocial considerations can also be introduced influencing the degree of perception, including sexuality, cultural expectations, privacy and religious issues.

For instance, if a patient is given well-meaning (but not necessarily correct) advice that his condition is serious (such as information from an MRI indicating 'degenerative changes'), this negative information will be attended to in the brain over other sensory information and can tend to increase the neural hypersensitivity. The pain is now produced by an overly sensitised neural system, which can have the effect of 'amplifying' or 'turning up' the pain.

Annoyingly, this pain can also be triggered by the merest, obtuse physical stimulation. This is known as a 'flare-up', and it is helpful for the patient to understand the perceived pain level does not necessarily reflect any extra structural damage. In fact, a 'flare-up' rarely reflects any extra structural damage.

It is important to recognise that chronic pain is not just acute pain with a longer duration. Chronic stress and pain cycles lower pain thresholds by depleting dopamine and elevating adrenaline, which in time, tightens already constricted and overloaded protective muscles. In fact, when the pain can't be controlled, panic sets in. The patients do not move; they stress about the pain and they catastrophise (imagine the 'worse-case' scenario). Perhaps a clinician has told them they have done very serious damage and need to rest. The pain is amplified.

Adopting poor posture patterns (particularly while sitting), inability to relax muscles, life stresses and lifestyle factors, sleep deficiency, hormonal shifts, depression, anxiety and dietary factors can also then disrupt normal pain modulation.

In fact, long-term pain has been shown to change the plasticity of the brain. It has long been clinically observed that once the nerve structure is altered because of irritation of any sort, the pain may persist even after the aggravating stimulus has been removed.

There is a favourite analogy for this effect. A lit match may start a kindling fire in the woods, which may progress eventually to become a roaring forest fire. Putting out the match too late (the cause) will not stop the raging forest fire. The forest fire will develop a life of its own and need to be controlled independently.

The same applies to the nervous system. The overstimulated nerve and its immediate neural system, therefore, is then said to become hypersensitive — a forest fire. This is called central sensitisation and plays a major role in maintaining ongoing chronic pain. Any small aggravation to this oversensitive nerve can now trigger off the pain cycle, often with 'overkill', — a flare-up — because of convergence between closely related nerves, often to many and varied regions.

It is not always possible to identify a particular nerve. In fact, small, unmyelinated nerve fibres are frequently responsible for this phenomenon, where functional (and measurable) changes may occur in the brain.

There are three criteria to diagnose chronic (or persistent or central sensitisation) pain. The first criterion entails the brain registering disproportionate pain. This implies that the severity of pain and related reported and perceived disability are disproportionate to the nature and extent of injury or pathology. The second criterion is the presence of diffuse pain distribution, allodynia (sensitive to touch, hot and cold), and hyperalgesia, (increased response to a painful stimulus), and thirdly, the hypersensitivity of senses unrelated to the musculoskeletal system (also called smudging).

When a nerve is pathologically compressed or entrapped, the nerve and its branches are subject to increased friction and stretch because they are unable to slide and glide normally in their sheaths. The smallest tension placed on any part of this now sensitive nerve will be dissipated in all directions, triggering and increasing the pain cycle.

Chronic pain can sensitize (and, in the process, confuse) the natural protective mechanisms of the brain, causing a chronically hyper-aroused system and magnifying the brain's perception of the pain.

A Word Here on Smudging

This process occurs mainly in the area of the brain within the cortex, often referred to as the *cortical homunculus* (literally, little man in the brain) — the brain's map of the body.

This is a neurological 'map' of the anatomical divisions of the body, which includes two types: sensory and motor. It really is a map of the proportionate association of the cortex with body members (hands, feet, back, sex organs etc.). It also reflects kinesthetic proprioception, the sense of the relative position of body parts during movement (See Figure 29).

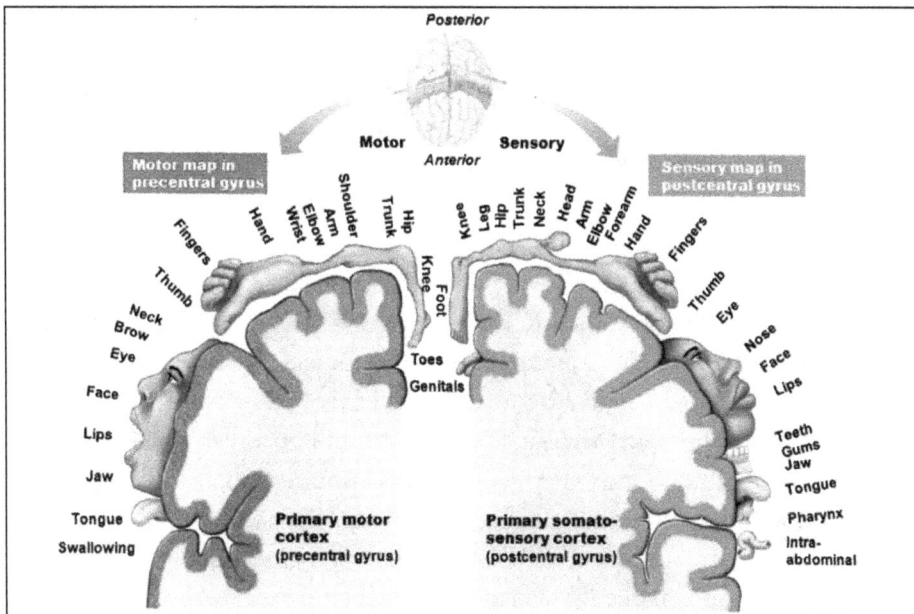

Figure 29. Body maps in the primary motor cortex and somatosensory cortex of the cerebrum

When a repetitive (overkill) message from the extremity is received in the cortical homunculus, not just one area fires up. As stated earlier, because of convergence between closely related nerves, instead of perhaps five percent of the brain being stimulated, other areas next to it are hijacked — up to twenty percent. This can affect and distort perception of thoughts, sensations, images, memories, movement and emotions. This effect is called *smudging* and can cause the brain to think this situation is as bad as what it has ever been, and, correspondingly, it is never going to 'get better', a catastrophysing reaction.

What may be considered a simple nerve injury may be magnified by the brain — the central nervous system (CNS) — so that a whole region may be involved. Certainly, there is a complete interaction where control of the immunological and endocrine systems may become abnormal. This can impact on emotional well-being, disability and widespread pain, so much so that a proportion of patients go on to develop chronic fatigue syndrome, fibromyalgia and immunological disorders.

This will quickly have an impact on the patient's mental health, causing them to lose concentration and focus. They will feel emotional and automatically react negatively to situations, which can lead to catastrophising, anxiety, depression, sleep disorders and affect their sexual health and relationships. The overall effect is debilitation.

In the case of pelvic dysfunction, patients presenting with pelvic pain symptoms may be experiencing a total level of pain from a number of contributors. These may include the joint injury, muscle spasm and associated regional myofascial trigger points, connective tissue adhesions and restrictions, neural compression, deficient pain modulators and stress, all complicated by a vicious pain cycle. Management of this situation relies on determining what the core problem is driving the entire complex — treating that, then tackling any residual and persistent pain cycle.

In the context of this book, it is advised, and has already been stated, it is important to initially assess the lumbar-pelvic region, in particular the sacroiliac joint, as being the probable source of the core problem — the match that triggers, and continues to trigger, the forest fire. (There are, of course, other joints and nerves that can trigger the fire and these should be assessed also.)

If pelvic dysfunction, or sacroiliac joint rotation (or other musculoskeletal condition) is found to be the correct underlying diagnosis, and if this is then treated, it is not uncommon to find that extreme nerve sensitivity and its complications may soon markedly decrease or completely resolve without further interventions. However, in some cases, even after treating the cause (the match) the resultant forest fire may still have to be addressed — the chronic or persistent pain scenario.

What is distressing is that with some patients, the majority of interventions such as blocks, stimulators and drugs, may eventually stop working. The neuro-plasticity of the brain has been changed to view this 'forest fire' state as a protective armament; it sees pain as 'good'.

This can be changed! A few words must be said about the emerging and interesting field of study concerning neuroplasticity. Neuroplasticity is loosely defined as the brain's ability to continually adapt to new information and expe-riences by changing its structure, function or chemistry. For example, changes such as a loss of white matter have been shown to occur in patients as a response to chronic pain. Now, research shows that relief of pain can reverse structural and functional changes and restore normal brain function.

Chronic Pain Management

For all cases of chronic pain cycles and neural hypersensitivity, there are a number of practical ways to decrease nerve sensitisation, i.e., to down-regulate an oversensitive nervous system.

- Education. Understanding the situation, an explanation of pain mecha-nisms, particularly the pitfalls of the recovery process in persistent pain. The patient must have ideas for taking control of recovery. Using edu-cational tools in the clinic to accurately explain pain reduces the threat of pain. This decreases the need for the body to over-engage other coping systems by bringing in the sympathetic, immune, endocrine and motor systems.

- Knowledge is power here. The patient will gain confidence from under-standing what pain is: to realise pain is an emotion; it is not visible but can be analysed. The patient may need to learn to accept that sometimes pain can't be easily 'cured', and must learn to manage it. This knowledge helps to reduce the perception of pain. Patients must learn to take responsibility for the pain and control how it is managed.

- In this regard, it is also important to understand that pain can lead to depression ('the blues'). This must be addressed as a depressed mood effectively shoots more messages to the brain, which is interpreted as more pain, setting off a vicious cycle. Education (and medication) as well as controlled exercise helps to break this pain cycle, so we should focus on mood as well as pain. By gradually re-engaging in normal activity, thereby getting more normal input into the brain, it is possible to begin to desensitise the hypersensitive pathways and normalise them. The following procedures can be helpful.

- Keeping active. Keeping active generally will promote recovery by:

  - Avoiding disuse effects of excessive rest

  - Regaining function and therefore, independence

  - Producing natural pain-relieving chemicals (endorphins)

  - Stimulating production of serotonin (the feel-good hormone)

  - Retraining the nervous system

- The following procedures can be helpful:

  - Gentle, rhythmic manual mobilising techniques have been found to ease pain.

  - Rhythmical and gentle exercise

  - Yoga

  - Feldenkrais. Feldenkrais has developed therapeutic exercises using sensation-based movements. These can be an effective basis for gentle introductory sensory-awareness routines.

  - Cardiovascular Exercise. There is well-documented evidence that aerobic exercise raises endorphin levels, which has the effect of decreasing pain. It also lowers a person's stress response, which assists in anxiety relief.

- Resistance Exercise. Weight training, Pilates, swimming

- Heat/ice application

- Cognitive Behavioural Therapy. Challenging maladaptive cognitive structures and processes, such as distraction activities, relaxation therapy and increased engagement with pleasurable activities

- Meditation. Can help with decreasing anxiety

- Mindfulness training. Learning awareness of thoughts, emotions and sensations. How we think and feel has a profound effect on all aspects of our physiology. When we are frustrated, angry, stressed, fearful, worried or depressed, everything — including pain — can seem worse.

- Positive thinking, affirmations. Patients may be able to learn to control and change their thoughts. Conversely, as thoughts are nerve impulses, negative thinking alone may drive persistent pain states.

- Guided imagery. Engages the power of the mind to reduce anxiety, depression and stress.

- Hypnosis
- Relaxation training. Many different techniques for this, including the Wise-Anderson Protocol, mentioned in the Introduction.
- Diet. What you eat has a direct and immediate effect on your hormone levels, mood, pain tolerance and energy levels. The Mediterranean Diet can be effective in this regard. Besides health benefits related to managing cardiovascular disease and cancers, this diet has been considered to produce a generalised anti-inflammatory effect.

  - Emphasise fruits, dark green leafy vegetables, whole grains, legumes, nuts, seeds.

  - Eat a rainbow of fruits and vegetables — orange, green, yellow, red, purple, white.

  - Choose low-glycaemic index (GI) carbohydrates — sweet potatoes, oats, wholegrain breads. Cut back on high GI carbohydrates (white breads, cakes, donuts, sugars etc.).

  - Essential fatty acids. Choose more omega-3 (anti-inflammatory) foods (walnuts, flax seeds, salmon, cherries, turmeric, dark green leafy vegetables, and soy). Choose less omega-6 and 9 (pro-inflammatory) foods (margarine, chips, cookies, cakes, biscuits, salad dressings, chocolate bars). However, dark chocolate has natural antioxidant properties, and it has also been shown to lower blood pressure — 2 squares after dinner, but only if it's 70 percent cocoa.

  - Resveratrol. Found in skin of grapes, blueberries and raspberries, green tea. Have red wine with dinner (one or two glasses).

  - Moderate use of yoghurt and low-fat cheese

  - Eat less meat and dairy.

  - If possible, all foods should be fresh, locally and organically grown.

- Electro-neuromodulation. This involves using electric current to modify pain perception. The most common and inexpensive method is transcutaneous electrical nerve stimulation (TENS). TENS may work through these mechanisms:

  - Prolonged stimulation causes the release of endorphins, resulting in a systemic analgesic effect.

  - Gate-close theory. Afferent nerve pathways are blocked, limiting the transference of messages to the brain that are interpreted as pain. A more scientific explanation is that by stimulating the large A-beta mechanosensory fibres, nociceptor transmission is inhibited at the dorsal horn of the spinal cord (the message that could be interpreted by the brain as pain is blocked here).

- If the person is given control of the TENS unit, this may increase their perceived control of their pain, reducing the threat value and anxiety associated with the pain, thus modulating the pain experience.

- Other methods of electro-neuromodulation are high galvanic electrotherapy (mild electric impulse) and pulsed radiofrequency (PRF). PRF delivers an electromagnetic field, which modifies neurocellular function with minimal cellular destruction. These procedures have documented varying degrees of success (up to 80% for pelvic pain and urgency).

- InterX. The interX is an electrical device that provides interactive stimulation. The modality uses high-amplitude, high-density stimulation to the cutaneous nerves, activating the body's natural pain relieving mechanisms.

- Acupuncture, dry needling

- Pain medication:

  - Simple analgesics — aspirin, paracetamol, tramadol

  - Anti-inflammatory drugs – NSAID

  - Pain modulators — work on neurogenic pain (gabapentin, Lyrica)

  - Antidepressants — tricyclics and other groups

  - Narcotics — to prevent constipation, morphine (Endone, oxycodone, naloxone + or –)

- Computed tomographic (CT)-guided pudendal nerve block techniques. There has been documentation of successful treatments by injecting the critical zone of compression of the pudendal nerve, mostly at the sacrospinous and sacrotuberous ligaments and the falciform process. The area is injected with lidocaine and long-release glucocorticoids.

- Botox injections into the suspected compressed areas

- Sensory pain. Because the pudendal nerve is a sensory nerve, it can produce sensory changes on the skin (redness, irritability, intolerance to tight clothes and certain cloth textures). If dermatological interventions fail, look for SIJ dysfunction. One hundred percent white cotton underwear can help the tissues to breathe more easily. Opt for organic tampons and choose 100 percent cotton pads for menstruation or urinary incontinence. Avoid other irritants like deodorant and certain soaps.

- Myofascial trigger point releases and deep tissue massage. As mentioned earlier, this concept is controversial and should be considered in context with the statement following below. Myofascial trigger points have been described as hyperirritable spots, usually within a taut band of skeletal muscle or the muscle's fascia. The spot is painful on compression and can give rise to a characteristic referred pain, tenderness and autonomic phenomenon. This spot can certainly contribute to the development of central sensitisation. Deep tissue massaging (and dry needling) has been found to be an effective treatment for reducing pain.

A Note of Caution About Myofascial Trigger Points

I have a cautionary message to deliver when treating 'trigger points' arising from an extremely oversensitive neuromuscular system. It is well-documented that patients with enhanced descending facilitation (persistent pain or central sensitisation) may be aggravated by hands-on techniques, for xample, manual therapy. Similarly, I have found that by applying over-vigorous or prolonged digital or manual treatments of any type can retrigger an already overreactive neural system, creating an even more complex pain cycle. I personally don't apply trigger point massages or even deep tissue massages to any pudendal neuralgia patient, although I concede, with care, it may be a useful technique.

Along these lines, as mentioned earlier, recent evidence would highlight that trigger points are a controversial phenomenon, an issue that will challenge our profession. In a keynote address at the International Pelvic Pain Society meeting in Chicago in 2015, renowned physiotherapy luminary Kari Bo stated research by Quinter et al., (Rheumatology 2014), that the construct of myofascial pain syndrome caused by trigger points remains conjecture. In fact, Quinter states that the theory can be discarded, a finding that Bo related specifically to chronic pelvic floor muscle spasm.

These statements have been challenged by other researchers (Dommerholt and Gerwin, J Bodyw Mov Ther 2015, and Fitzgerald et al., J Urol, 09-13) and certainly anecdotal evidence suggests that this technique should not be laid to rest.

In fact, we should be mindful of the comments of another physiotherapy luminary, Lorimer Moseley (2017), who said that he considers that there are very few, if any, physiotherapy treatments where there is a lot of research to say it has no effect. What the research does say is that the effect that it seems to have may not be mediated by the mechanisms we thought it was mediated by.

A Note of Caution About Pelvic Floor Exercises

For the same reason, I am also very careful when prescribing pelvic floor exercises. The pudendal nerve supplies most of the pelvic floor muscles, which includes the urinary and anal sphincters. (The deep muscles are supplied directly from the sacral plexus.) As these muscles (and sphincters) may also be in a chronic protective spasm cycle (set off by any cause irritating the pudendal nerve) and be hypersensitive themselves, I have found aggressive pelvic floor exercises (and some other pelvic, lower-back and abdominal exercises) can often trigger and maintain neural pain cycles. This is reinforced by Jerome Weiss's[1] warning: Any compression to an inflamed nerve (either by exercises or massage) not only can cause local pain, but also creates increased muscle tension, which is transferred to the penetrating organs (urethra, vagina, scrotum and rectum).

In fact, in most of these cases, the reverse is needed — targeted relaxation techniques and relaxation training sessions of the pelvic floor muscles may be more beneficial.

Finally, it is worthwhile reminding patients of this hopeful statement by Pearson[2], who presents a well-formed explanation of the ability of patients with persistent pain to return to normal function:

> Remember, all these things that the nervous system has learned can be changed back. Neurons can become less sensitive; they can stop paying attention to and stop misinterpreting normal sensation as dangerous. Sensors can change back to the way they were; the map of the body on the brain can go back to its normal state and the muscles can regain their normal coordinated action. All it took was the wrong circumstances and lots of practice to get them to act the way they are. Now the patient has to practice new things. With Patience, Persistence, Compassion and Practice the patient will find ways to change them back, instead of just covering up the pain.

Introduction

1. Treede, R.D., Jensen, T.S. Campbell, J.N., Cruccu, G., Dostrovsky, J.O. et al. (2008). Neuropathic pain. Redefinition and a grading system for clinical and research purposes. *Neurology*, April 29, Vol.70, No 18 1630-1635.

2. Labat, J.J. et al. (1990). *Journal d'Urologie* 96 (5) 239-44.

3. Labat, J.J. et al. (2007). *Neurology and Urodynamics*. DOI 10.1002/nau

4. Filler, A.G. (2009). Diagnosis and treatment of Pudendal Nerve Entrapment Syndromes Subtypes: Imaging, injections, and minimal access surgery. *Neurosurg Focus 26 (2):E92.* 1

5. Weiss, J.M. 2003. Presented at the International Pelvic Pain Society, 10th Scientific meeting on Chronic Pelvic Pain in Alberta, Canada, August 2003.

6. Prendergast, S.A., & Rummer, E.H. (2006). The Role of Physical Therapy in Treatment of Pudendal Neuralgia. The International Pelvic Pain Society. *Vision*. Vol. 15. No. 1.

7. Wise, D. & Anderson, R (2008). *A Headache in the Pelvis*. 5th Edition Published by National Centre for Pelvic Pain Research. PO Box 54, Occidental Ca, 95465.

8. Anderson, R.U., Wise, D. , Sawyer, T. , Chan T. (2005). Integration of myofascial trigger point release and paradoxical relaxation training treatment of chronic pelvic pain in men. *Journal of Urology*, Jul;174(1):155-60.

9. Muller, R. Gertz, K.J. Molton, I.R. Terrill A.L. (2016). Effects of a Tailored positive psychology intervention on well-being and pain in individuals with chronic pain and a physical disability: A feasibility trial. *Clin J Pain*, 32(1): 32-44

10. Mathias, S.D. et al. (1996). *Obstet Gynacol.* 87:321-327.

11. Roberts, R.D. et al. (1997). A review of clinical and pathological prostatitis syndrome. *Urology*, 49:809-821

12. Dornan, P.R. Coppieters, M. (2012). A musculoskeletal approach for patients with pudendal neuralgia: A cohort study. *BJUI*, Oct.

Chapter 1

1. Lee, D. (2011). The Pelvic Girdle. Fourth Edition. P61. Elsevier.

2. Jacob, H.A.C, Kissling, R.D. (1995). The mobility of the sacroiliac joints in healthy volunteers between 20 and 50 years of age, *Clin. Biomech.* (Bristol, Avon) 10(7) 352

3. Maigne, R. (1980). Low back pain of thorocolumbar origin. *Arch, Phys.Med.*Rehabil.61, 389–395

4. Maigne, R. (1981). Le Syndrome de la charmiere dorso-lombaire. Lombalgus basses, douleurs pseudo-viscerales, pseudo-douleurs de hanche, pseudo-tendinite des adducteurs. *Sem.Hop.* Paris. 57,11–12,545–554

Chapter 2

1. Hesch, J. (2011). Presented at the IPPS Workshop, Las Vegas.NV

2. Maitland, G.D. (2005). *Maitlands Vertebral Manipulation*, 7th ed. Philadelphia, PA. Elsevier.

Chapter 3

1. Weiss, J.M. (2003). presented at the International pelvic Pain Society 10th Scientific Meeting, on Chronic Pelvic Pain in Alberta, Canada.

2. Pearson, N. (2007). *Understand Pain, Live Well Again.* Penticton, British Columbia, Canada, Life is Now.

Further Reading

Explain Pain. David Butler and Lorimer Mosely. Norgroup Publications, Adelaide. S.Australia. (August 2010 Reprint)

Heal Pelvic Pain. Amy Stein. McGraw Hill. New York. 2009

Pelvic Pain Explained: What everyone needs to know. Stephanie Prendergast and Elizabeth H Rummer. Bowman & Littlefield, Maryland 2016.

Endometriosis and Pelvic Pain, (3rd Ed.). Susan Evans and Deborah Bush. Published by Dr Susan Evans, SA 2016.

So you've got pelvic pain ... Here's how to manage it.

www.ingramcontent.com/pod-product-compliance
Lightning Source LLC
Chambersburg PA
CBHW082111210326
41599CB00033B/6668